Volume 27

DECISION IN CHILD CARE

DECISION IN CHILD CARE
A Study of Prediction in Fostering

R. A. PARKER

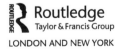

Routledge
Taylor & Francis Group

LONDON AND NEW YORK

First published in 1966 by George Allen & Unwin Ltd.

This edition first published in 2022
by Routledge
4 Park Square, Milton Park, Abingdon, Oxon OX14 4RN
605 Third Avenue, New York, NY 10017

Routledge is an imprint of the Taylor & Francis Group, an informa business

British Library Cataloguing in Publication Data
A catalogue record for this book is available from the British Library

ISBN: 978-1-03-203381-5 (Set)
ISBN: 978-1-00-321681-0 (Set) (ebk)
ISBN: 978-1-03-206813-8 (Volume 27) (hbk)
ISBN: 978-1-03-206818-3 (Volume 27) (pbk)
ISBN: 978-1-00-320399-5 (Volume 27) (ebk)

DOI: 10.4324/9781003203995

Publisher's Note
The publisher has gone to great lengths to ensure the quality of this reprint but points out that some imperfections in the original copies may be apparent.

Disclaimer
The publisher has made every effort to trace copyright holders and would welcome correspondence from those they have been unable to trace.

DECISION IN CHILD CARE

A STUDY OF PREDICTION IN FOSTERING

BY

R. A. PARKER

with a Foreword by

D. V. DONNISON

*Professor of Social Administration
in the University of London*

London

GEORGE ALLEN & UNWIN LTD

RUSKIN HOUSE   MUSEUM STREET

FIRST PUBLISHED IN 1966

SECOND IMPRESSION 1969

© *George Allen & Unwin Ltd., 1966*

SBN 04 362016 7

PRINTED IN GREAT BRITAIN
by Photolithography
UNWIN BROTHERS LIMITED
WOKING AND LONDON

ACKNOWLEDGEMENTS

I WOULD like to express my thanks to a number of people who have generously given assistance and advice in the course of this study. I am indebted to the Children's Committee of the Kent County Council for allowing me to conduct the research in their area and to have access to the necessary case records. In particular I would like to thank the Children's Officer, Miss D. E. Harvie, and the many members of the department who gave me a great deal of help.

I am very grateful too for the advice and help given me throughout this study by Professor D. V. Donnison and for the encouragement of Professor R. M. Titmuss. I have also appreciated the advice of Mr L. T. Wilkins and Dr M. H. Quenouille in regard to the statistical aspects of the enquiry. Robin Huws Jones read the draft and amongst other things, helped me to avoid including several passages which were not clear. Of course I alone am responsible for any shortcomings or inaccuracies which may appear in the book.

The research would never have been completed had it not been for the aid of a generous grant from the Sir Halley Stewart Trust and for this I am especially grateful. They have also contributed generously to part of the cost of publication. Thanks are also due to the London School of Economics who awarded me a research bursary; to the University of London Central Research Fund and the department of Social Administration at the School of Economics for grants for certain specific expenses.

FOREWORD

———

BY PROFESSOR D. V. DONNISON

IT has for years been said that social work cannot develop effectively and humanely—let alone claim the status due to a responsible profession—until a more systematic and reliable body of knowledge has been accumulated about its working methods, its achievements and its guiding principles. The research so far carried out in this field consists mainly of historical narratives dealing with particular branches of the profession, general surveys describing particular services or districts, and case studies of various kinds. Informative, perceptive and thought-provoking though much of it has been, a more careful selection of 'strategic' research questions and more rigorous analyses of accumulated experience will be required before social workers can be given the help which they have a right to expect from research.

It has also been said for years that social workers already possess within their files a rich store of experience and observation that could be of enormous value to their profession and to social scientists generally. But research workers have seldom made effective use of this material. Often lacking first-hand knowledge of social work, they have generally preferred to start from scratch with inquiries of their own rather than dig deep into the records.

More recently it has become fashionable to say that the problems to be studied in this field are so complex that they can only be effectively explored by full-time, inter-disciplinary teams of highly qualified specialists, backed by the generous funds that such operations demand.

It is against this background that Dr. Parker's study assumes a pioneering stature. He asks a basic question which social workers up and down the country must every day endeavour to answer: what are the factors that go to make a successful placing for a foster child? He examines the answers that others have given to this question, but deliberately adopts no assumptions or hypotheses of his own. Thanks to the help of the Kent County Children's Department, he then brings to bear on this question all the evidence available in this authority's files. In the course of the sophisticated analysis that follows, he shows how the outcome of a foster home placement can be predicted, demolishes a number of popular illusions, and considers the implications of his findings. He insists throughout that research can never replace the skill and judgement of those who must actually take decisions about foster children and assume responsibility for their welfare. But it can furnish them with the lessons to be derived from a mass of experience far greater than one person could accumulate, and pose more clearly the questions which can be answered only with the aid of a trained and sensitive judgement.

Dr. Parker would be the first to remind us that his study deals only with one aspect of one field of social work, and takes our knowledge of it only a short step forward. But the example he sets is an impressive one, which can be followed by others—virtually single-handed, like himself—without waiting for the more massive resources that will also be required in this field.

CONTENTS

CONTENTS

1

INTRODUCTION

I

THE STUDY OF FOSTER CARE

A N important feature in the development of the child care service over the last fifteen years has been the emphasis placed upon boarding-out. In an atmosphere of statutory encouragement and Home Office enthusiasm local authorities have increasingly sought to place the children in their care with suitable foster parents. Indeed, the foster home has come to be regarded as the best way, other than adoption, of providing for the needs of the child who for one reason or another cannot remain in his own home.

Notwithstanding the apparent desirability and humanity of such a policy it ought, like any other, to be regarded as an experiment which needs to be observed and tested.[1] Neither the policy nor the practice of child placement can develop intelligently without reference to what is happening and has happened in a variety of foster homes throughout the country. The modification of existing policies, the formulation of new ones, and the improvement of social work techniques all depend upon the accessibility of past experience. Little opportunity, however, seems to have been taken since the implementation of the Children Act, 1948, to assess the policies which have been adopted or to assemble and make available the store of experience which has been accumulating.

---

[1] As Prof. D. V. Glass has pointed out—'Given a new service it is surely necessary to include as an integral part of the structure some provision for examining the results and ascertaining how far and as a result of which specific measure, the desired ends are being achieved'. ('The Application of Social Research'. *British Journal of Sociology*. Vol. 1, No. 1, March 1950, p. 23).

This study, which was carried out in Kent with the co-operation of the Children's Committee and the staff of the Children's Department, had as its aim these two objectives. That is, first, to assess the degree to which boarding-out has been successful, and second, to bring together and sift some of the recorded experience with a view to providing a basis upon which improvements in foster home placement might be made.

II

BACKGROUND TO THE CHILD CARE SERVICE

The child care service today[1] derives its form primarily from the Children Act of 1948. The three immediate antecedents of this Act are commonly considered to have been the correspondence in *The Times* during the summer of 1944,[2] particularly the letter from Lady Allen of Hurtwood; the case of Dennis O'Neill[3] who died in a foster home where ill-treatment was subsequently proved; and lastly the Curtis and Clyde Committees which in 1946 published their findings on the care of deprived and homeless children in England and Wales, and Scotland respectively.[4] A fairly full examination of these influences, their detail and effect is provided in the Sixth Report of the Work of the Children's

---

[1] For an historical account of services for deprived children see J. S. Heywood, *Children in Care*. Routledge & Kegan Paul, 1959.

[2] Various issues July 15, 1944 onwards. Lady Allen opening the correspondence on July 15 claimed that 'the public are, for the most part, unaware that many thousands of children are being brought up under repressive conditions that are generations out of date and are unworthy of our traditional care of children' adding that 'because no one government department is responsible the problem is the more difficult to tackle,' but concluding that 'a public inquiry, with full government support, is urgently needed to explore this largely uncivilized territory.' Considerable correspondence followed this letter. By the end of the month nineteen letters had appeared. Susan Isaacs wrote (18th) and so did George Bernard Shaw (July 21st and August 2nd), and many others. With but a few exceptions all agreed in essence with Lady Allen's letter and called for an inquiry. For example: 'We need a comprehensive study of the situation in all its aspects and based on this an equally comprehensive reform.' (Gwendolen Chester—July 19th).

[3] See 'Report on the Circumstances which led to the Boarding-out of Dennis and Terence O'Neill at Bank Farm, Minsterley, and the steps taken to supervise their Welfare.' Cmd. 6636. May 1945, (The Monckton Report). An awareness of such dangers was certainly not new however: for instance the 20th Annual Report of the Ministry of Health (1938–9. Cmd. 6089) stressed that the arrangements for visiting foster children were often inadequate, adding that these were 'strikingly illustrated by the fact that a case of ill-treatment of a boarded-out child was discovered by the local officer of the N.S.P.C.C.' (p. 72).

[4] Cmd. 6922 'Report of the Care of Children Committee', 1946. (Curtis) and Cmd. 6911 'Report of the Committee on Homeless Children.' (Clyde).

Department of the Home Office[1] and need not be discussed here.

Briefly the Act places central responsibility for the care of children deprived of a normal home life on the Home Office. The local authorities however are responsible for its implementation, and the children for whom they provide care are those received under section 1 of the Act and those committed to their care as a 'fit person' by a juvenile court under the provisions of the 1933 and 1963 Children and Young Persons Acts. There are thus two main channels through which children 'come into care',[2] but in each case they become the responsibility of the children's departments[3] set up under the Children Act.

The Act itself places a duty on local authorities 'to receive into care, where it appears to them in the interests of the welfare of the child, any child in their area under the age of 17 years who has no parent or guardian, or is abandoned or lost, or whose parents or guardians are prevented for the time being, or permanently, by incapacity or any other circumstances from providing for his proper accommodation, maintenance and upbringing.'[4] Not only do local authorities have this duty to receive such children into their care, but also to return them to their parents or guardians whenever this is reasonable and possible. If this is not achieved the child stays in care until the age of 18.

The Children Act, 1948, does not give an authority power to take a child into care against the wishes of his parents. It provides, in effect, for a voluntary agreement between parent and authority. However, once a child has been received into care under this provision the children's committee can in certain circumstances pass a resolution assuming parental rights (section 2 of the Act). Such decisions are not taken lightly and machinery exists to safe-

[1] Home Office Sixth Report of the Work of the Children's Department May, 1951. pp. 3–6 (henceforth often referred to as the 'Sixth Report').

[2] Children can also be accepted into care under section 6 (4) of the 1948 Children Act, that is from an Approved School, viz. 'A child on licence from an Approved School or under supervision of the managers, who has no home or whose home appears to be unsatisfactory.' (6th Report para. 23, p. 7.) Few children are received under this provision—in 1950 there were 36 in England and Wales, and 68 in the year ending March 31, 1960. Recently too under Section 5 (1) of the Matrimonial Proceedings (Children) Act, 1958, and under section 2 (1) of the Matrimonial Proceedings (Magistrates' Courts) Act, 1960, a small number of children have been taken into care: in the year ending March 31, 1963 a total of 117.

[3] The responsible body at local level is, of course, the Children's Committee of the Council.

[4] Sixth Report para. 24, p. 7.

guard the rights of the parents.[1] These resolutions are usually passed when the child is abandoned, orphaned, and sometimes when the parent or parents are suffering from a permanent disability or where they are unfit by their 'habits or mode of life' to have care of the child.

Under the Children and Young Persons Acts, 1933 and 1963, juvenile courts can make a fit person order in respect of a child brought before them either as delinquent or as in need of care, protection, or control.[2] The vast majority of such orders commit the child to the care of a local authority which acts as the fit person. Those in need of care, protection or control,[3] are children 'against whom certain offences have been committed, including children neglected, abandoned, exposed, assaulted, or ill-treated in a manner likely to cause unnecessary suffering or injury to health; children, who through lack of proper care or guardianship, have fallen into bad associations or have been exposed to moral danger; children who have failed to attend school regularly, and children beyond control'.[4]

About a quarter of the children committed to the care of the local authorities by the courts are delinquent.[5] These are usually those who, in the opinion of the court, need to be removed from their home influence but do not require approved school or other types of residential training.

For whatever reason the court makes a fit person order committing a child to the care of the local authority, such an order

---

[1] 'The rights of parents are safeguarded by the provision in the Children Act which enables a parent to object to the passing of a resolution. The lodging of an objection, on the receipt of the notice that the local authority is required to give the parent, has the effect of referring the issue to a juvenile court for determination. In addition, a parent may apply to a juvenile court at any time for an order bringing a resolution to an end' (7th Report of the Work of the Children's Department, Home Office 1955, para. 87, p. 19). In England and Wales the number of resolutions in force on November 30, 1954 was 9,648, which represented almost 15 per cent of all the children in care on that date and just over 20 per cent of all children received into care under the Children Act (7th Report, para. 84, p. 19). By March 31, 1960 this figure had changed little—9,752 and the proportions were approximately 12 per cent and 23 per cent respectively (8th Report, 1961, p. 101, table 1).

[2] By the Children and Young Persons (Amendment) Act, 1952, the definition of a child in need of care or protection was extended to include cases where the neglect was not wilful, i.e. through ignorance, low mental capacity, and so on.

[3] This is dealt with in sections 61–64 of the 1933 Act. Sections 61 and 64 however have now been repealed by the 1963 Act, and replaced by new sections (2 and 3).

[4] Sixth Report, para. 34, p. 10.

[5] In 1954 of those received under a fit person order, about 33 per cent were offenders (7th Report, p. 154). By 1960 the proportion had dropped somewhat to 27 per cent (8th Report, p. 102).

remains in operation until the child reaches the age of 18. However, orders can be terminated before this if upon application a revocation is granted by the court. Sometimes a child is returned home to his parents (without the order having been revoked) 'on trial' at the discretion of the fit person.

Thus of the two legal structures by which a child can be received into care one is voluntary and the other obligatory. Once in care however the child may be looked after in a number of ways which are not determined by such legal considerations. One of these methods is placement in a foster home supervised by a children's department. It is this form of care with which the study is concerned.

III

THE DEVELOPMENT OF FOSTER CARE

The official use of foster care is no new idea. Indeed at the beginning of this century some 7,350 children were boarded-out by the Poor Law authorities in England and Wales. Until the late thirties, however, it remained undeveloped as a means of caring for children deprived of a normal home life. It seems to have been mainly a residual form of care restricted to orphans, deserted children and others who were unlikely to be reunited with their own families. Most children continued to be looked after in institutions of one kind or another.[1]

Probably the most significant change in the pre-war period came with the 1933 Children and Young Persons Act which

[1] A sample of figures drawn from the Annual Reports of the Local Government Board and later the Ministry of Health (29th Annual Report of the Local Government Board 1899–1900 Cd. 292; 39th Annual Report of the Local Government Board 1909–10 Cd. 5260, Part I; 1st Annual Report of the Ministry of Health 1919–20 Cmd. 932, Part III; 10th Annual Report of the Ministry of Health 1928–9 Cmd. 3362, Part III; 20th Annual Report of the Ministry of Health 1938–9 Cmd. 6089, Part III) give some indication of the extent of the boarding-out work of poor law authorities in the first forty years of this century.

Children 'in Care' of Poor Law Authorities in England and Wales

As at: January 1	Boarded-out No.	%	In Institutions Without Parents No.	%	Total No.	%
1900	7,358	18·4	32,710	81·6	40,068	100
1910	8,813	19·7	35,999	80·3	44,812	100
1920	9,354	13·6	59,283	86·4	68,637	100
1929	8,328	12·6	57,797	87·4	66,125	100
1939	6,281	15·7	33,617	84·3	39,898	100

obliged local authorities, with certain exceptions, to board-out children who were committed to their care.[1] In spite of this however neither the total number nor the proportion of children placed in foster homes by local authorities in England and Wales was greater in 1939 than it was in 1900.

By 1946 however there had been a rapid expansion. In that year the Curtis Committee reported that 13,900 children were boarded-out by local authorities—representing about 28 per cent of all those for whom they were responsible.[2] Three years later the new child care service had increased this to 19,271 or 35 per cent[3] and today the number stands at 31,208 or 51 per cent[4]. These bare figures represent a sweeping change in social policy with regard to children in care.[5] Doubtless this was partly a consequence of evacuation schemes and of post-war reforming zeal but there appear to have been other important and inter-related factors which were influential.

First, there was a growing recognition of the disadvantages and deficiencies of institutional care. This led to various improvements being made: equally important it led to foster care, as the only other practicable alternative, being viewed in a favourable light. Second, certain conclusions in the psychological field were gradually presented and widely accepted.[6] These stressed the vital role which the relationship between mother and child plays in mental health and social development and had obvious implications for child care policy. If the child was deprived of this natural relationship, then the best substitute was likely to be provided by

[1] See Curtis Report Cmd. 6922 para. 48, p. 15. There were probably about 550 fit person order cases boarded-out by local authorities in England and Wales in 1939 (Estimate based upon information in 5th Report of the Work of the Children's Branch, Home Office, 1938.) This figure had risen to 6,000 in 1946 (Curtis report, p. 18).

[2] Ibid. Estimated from Table IV, p. 27, i.e. addition of categories 1, 2, and 6. (4,900 P.A. children; 3,000 homeless evacuees, and 6,000 F.P.O. cases.) Percentage based upon total of approximately 50,000 deduced from the same table.

[3] Sixth Report, May 1951, table 1, p. 148.

[4] Home Office Children in Care in England and Wales, March 1963, Cmnd. 2240. p. 5.

[5] In Scotland boarding-out had been developed earlier and more extensively. The Clyde Committee, for instance, unlike its English counterpart merely re-emphasized the value of good foster care ('boarding-out with good foster parents should remain the principal method of dealing with the homeless child', para. 45, p. 15). From figures given for 1945 in the second appendix to this report it could be deduced that there were 8,650 children who might have been regarded as 'in care' as defined by the subsequent Children Act, 6,450 of whom were boarded-out—75 per cent. Before the war the proportion if anything was slightly higher. In recent years it has remained at about the 60 per cent level.

[6] e.g. John Bowlby's Maternal Care and Mental Health. W.H.O. 1951.

a foster mother. Third, and closely related to this, short-term as well as long-term foster care came to be seen as both possible and desirable. This increased its scope considerably. Fourth, the lack of sufficient adequate residential accommodation in a situation of rapidly growing demand and severe building restrictions placed a premium on foster care.

There was a further reason which helps to explain the ease with which this policy was adopted: the happy coincidence that the most desirable provision was for once the most economical. For instance, after stressing the value of boarding-out for the child a Home Office circular pointed out that 'expansion of boarding-out should relieve pressure on accommodation in children's homes and residential nurseries, at a time when restrictions on capital investment limit severely the improvement of existing premises. . . . Finally boarding-out is the least expensive method of child care both in money and manpower, and in the present financial condition of the country it is imperative to exercise the strictest economy consistent with a proper regard for the interests of the children.[1] It continues to cost child care organizations considerably less to keep a child in a foster home than in a children's home or nursery. If, for example, the proportion of children boarded-out by local authorities in England and Wales was increased from 52 per cent to 75 per cent, then on the basis of recent figures this would represent a saving of at least £4¾ million each year—nearly a quarter of the total annual public expenditure on the whole child care service.[2]

The interplay and effect of these influences can be seen in the well-known reports of the Curtis and Clyde Committees, and in the statutory requirement of the Children Act for local authorities to board-out whenever possible.[3] They can also be recognized in numerous other reports, memoranda and circulars which in

[1] Home Office, Circular H.O. 258/52. November 1952, para. 2.
[2] See Home Office *Children in Care in England and Wales*, March 1962, Cmnd. 1876, Table III, p. 10. The financial incentive has not declined as more children are boarded-out. In 1952–3 for instance (Cmd. 9154—*Children in Care of Local Authorities*, 1953) to raise the level of boarding-out from 42 per cent to 75 per cent would have represented a 27 per cent saving in the total cost of the service (i.e. a saving of £3,635,308 in a service costing £13,416,428). Likewise the average cost of institutional care per child in 1952–3 was 2·9 times that of the boarded-out child—by 1961–2 this ratio was 3·7. Between 1952–3 and 1961–2 the cost of foster care per child week rose 145 per cent; the average cost of a child in a home rose 183 per cent.
[3] Children Act, 1948, Section 13 (1) (a).

their turn sought to encourage its expansion.[1] For instance, the value of foster care was stressed as early as 1946 in a joint memorandum from the Home Office and Ministry of Health. This pointed out that 'the great advantage of boarding-out in a good foster home over other forms of care is that it not only provides a child with the individual affection, and stable personal relationships of a real home, but it is also the most natural preparation for adult life. The foster child, growing up as a member of a family, can see and respond to the demands which family life makes on the individual members, and becomes aware of some of the ordinary difficulties of life, and the ways in which people meet them'.[2]

The Select Committee on Estimates which reported on the child care service in 1952 seems to have been particularly influential. It emphasized, for instance, that 'local authorities are under a specific obligation to use boarding-out as the normal method of providing for children in their care with an implied obligation to give it an overriding priority and to make it the main objective of all their work in this connection'.[3] The minutes of this Committee, for example, record that the Chairman asked the Children's Officer of the London County Council 'what sort of prodding does the Home Office give local authorities about boarding-out?' and was told 'they are always on about it'.[4] In their departmental reply to this report the Home Office claimed that they were 'at one with the Committee in wanting to secure a large expansion of boarding-out and to see this achieved in all suitable cases, bearing in mind that expansion cannot be forced unduly without risk of unsuitable placings and consequent damage to the children'[5] and added in a recommendation, that they should 'issue renewed

[1] Although as Jean Heywood has pointed out in her book *Children in Care*, in the very early days of the new service 'the immediate provision of shelter and care became the overriding anxiety, accentuated by lack of staff. In this situation local authorities turned their attention, not to the providing of field staff . . . but the provision of the right kind of residential care and the improvement of its quality' (p. 161).

[2] Memorandum on the Boarding-out of Children and Young Persons 1946, p. 3.

[3] Sixth Report from the Select Committee on Estimates, Session 1951–2 (Child Care), House of Commons Paper 235, para. 14, p. xiv.

[4] Ibid., para. 587, p. 45 (n.b. in 1952 the L.C.C. rate of boarding-out was 25 per cent, so that the reply might not be completely typical).

[5] Departmental reply to the Sixth Report from the Select Committee on Estimates, Session 1951–2 (Child Care), Appendix 1 to the 13th Report of the Select Committee on Estimates 1951–2. H.C. 328. Also published and circulated to local authorities as a memorandum by the Home Office together with circular 258/52.

instructions to local authorities to the effect that boarding-out is, with due safeguards, the primary objective'.[1]

However, it must not be concluded that the various local authorities pursued this policy in exactly the same way. Some were more cautious than others; some faced different local traditions and different attitudes towards fostering, whilst some had better opportunities for recruiting foster mothers than others.[2] Because the Home Office has continually emphasized the policy it does not follow that individual children's committees of the County Councils and County Borough Councils have accepted it blindly, ignoring local conditions and their own beliefs and attitudes. Rates of boarding-out vary considerably between authorities and bear witness to this. For example in England and Wales in 1952 the highest rate was 82 per cent and the lowest 20 per cent and in 1963 100 per cent and 28 per cent.[3]

Nevertheless there is substantial evidence that the foster home is regarded throughout the country as an integral and important feature of child care policy. There is also some evidence to support the contention that in many cases the good foster home is preferable to residential care.[4] However, although the existence of the policy is clear and it can claim many persuasive advocates there has been little attempt to assess its success.

IV

THE LACK OF CRITICAL ASSESSMENT

The proportion of children in the care of local authorities in England and Wales who are boarded-out has risen from 35 per cent in 1949 to 52 per cent in 1963, and in absolute terms from 19,271 to 31,208.[5] A growing number of foster home placements however does not in itself indicate an increasingly successful policy. To judge this it is necessary to know the proportion which was successful. This fact seems to have been given some recog-

---

[1] Ibid., recommendation 2, p. 2.
[2] For example, in Scotland there has been a tradition of foster care over a long period on which the requirements of the Children Act could successfully be superimposed.
[3] See *Children in Care in England and Wales*, 1952 (Cmd. 8910), and 1963 (Cmnd. 2240).
[4] The most influential evidence has been collected by Bowlby in his W.H.O. monograph *Maternal Care and Mental Health*, 1951.
[5] See Appendix 1.

ACKNOWLEDGEMENTS

I WOULD like to express my thanks to a number of people who have generously given assistance and advice in the course of this study. I am indebted to the Children's Committee of the Kent County Council for allowing me to conduct the research in their area and to have access to the necessary case records. In particular I would like to thank the Children's Officer, Miss D. E. Harvie, and the many members of the department who gave me a great deal of help.

I am very grateful too for the advice and help given me throughout this study by Professor D. V. Donnison and for the encouragement of Professor R. M. Titmuss. I have also appreciated the advice of Mr L. T. Wilkins and Dr M. H. Quenouille in regard to the statistical aspects of the enquiry. Robin Huws Jones read the draft and amongst other things, helped me to avoid including several passages which were not clear. Of course I alone am responsible for any shortcomings or inaccuracies which may appear in the book.

The research would never have been completed had it not been for the aid of a generous grant from the Sir Halley Stewart Trust and for this I am especially grateful. They have also contributed generously to part of the cost of publication. Thanks are also due to the London School of Economics who awarded me a research bursary; to the University of London Central Research Fund and the department of Social Administration at the School of Economics for grants for certain specific expenses.

increasing attention is being given by local authorities to making
sure, as far as possible, that these do not occur'.[1]

Those working in this field are certainly striving to reduce the
number of foster home failures, but there is little to which they
can turn for guidance. There is a great deal of literature on related
topics, such as casework theory and practice, the psychology of
the family, the etiology and manifestations of maladjustment and
so on. This, though often useful, is not specific. To be of direct
use much of it has to be 'translated' to the problem of foster care,
and although there are certain similarities the result does not
always seem appropriate; for instance, the foster family is not an
ordinary family; nor do theories of sibling relationships necessarily apply to foster sibling relationships.

The little material available which is specifically concerned with
the problem is primarily of one type: namely the individual case
study, or the book or article woven around such studies. Simon
strongly criticized this situation in the USA in 1950. 'What we
have', he claimed, 'running through the entire literature [of child
placement] are statements of belief presented as theory, docu-
mented with cases. Or else certain points are made and illustrated
to enlighten the reader without measure or estimates as to validity
or reliability'.[2] The situation may have changed somewhat in
America; in this country the comment could stand today as an
accurate summary. Child care workers undertaking placements
have an increasing body of casework theory and training to help
them, but innumerable questions remain which such theory cannot
adequately answer.

Apart from their use as techniques in the practice of social work,
case study methods serve two other purposes well. First, they can
suggest hypotheses to be tested and studied; and second, they can
illustrate a theory or conclusion once it has been established. What
they are ill-equipped to do, and this appears to be the point Simon
is making, is to validate theories or ideas. For any theory or
generalization to be of practical value it must necessarily stand
the test of repeated application. Such a test cannot be provided by

[1] Seventh Report of the Work of the Children's Department, Home Office, 1955,
para. 37, p. 10.
[2] Abraham J. Simon 'Social and Psychological Factors in Child Placement'. *American
Journal of Orthopsychiatry*. April 1950, Vol. XX, No. 2, p. 293.

the case study approach, for by definition, it deals too intensively with each individual case to encompass such a wide review. It is probably because of this that caseworkers cannot always place sufficient confidence in the practical propositions which are found in contemporary child care literature and teaching.

There are two large gaps in our knowledge about child placement in particular. The success of the policy itself has never been critically examined; and the range of reliable information available to those who put the policy into practice is sadly limited. The emphasis in this study was primarily on filling the second of these. Its object was to provide information in such a way that it could be used as one means of reducing the number of foster home breakdowns. In doing this it also became possible to make a more general assessment of boarding-out in one area.

2

THE DEVELOPMENT OF THE STUDY

I

THE CONCEPT AND VALUE OF PREDICTION

BOARDING-OUT can, in a simplified form, be regarded as a two stage process. First there is the decision to make the placement and second, the subsequent supervision and casework help.[1] If the proportion of successful placements is to be increased improvements must be made at either one or both of these stages.

Logically the decision stage comes first and it predetermines to a large extent the supervision stage.[2] It includes the recruitment of foster parents, the selection of children suitable for boarding-out and any attempt at 'matching'. It is a complex process which once completed sets certain limits to what can be achieved in the future. Good casework supervision after a placement has been made can offer much but it cannot entirely overcome the consequences of a poor placing decision. Hence, of the two stages, that of the initial placement decision is the more fundamental and influential.

Since the scope of the research had to be limited it was decided to focus on this first stage of the boarding-out process, aiming to contribute towards the improvement of placing decisions. Although this problem can be approached in a number of ways it seemed most appropriate to treat it as one of making accurate predictions; for this is what any decision obliges us to do.

[1] The useful concept of this two-stage division in the boarding-out situation was suggested by a discussion of administrative decision-making in H. A. Simon's *Administrative Behaviour* (2nd edition) Macmillan, New York, 1961.
[2] cf. 'If the best use is to be made of the boarding-out system we are convinced that the initial placing of the child must be regarded as a matter of supreme importance, and very careful thought given to it by those responsible. . . . ' Report of the Boarding-Out Committee of the Scottish Advisory Council on Child Care, 1950, para. 6, p. 5.

Predictions are made on the basis of experience. Better predictions, and hence better decisions, can only be made by taking account of wider and more systematic knowledge of past events. Techniques have in fact been devised which enable this to be done. Basically they involve collecting information about numerous previous cases and analysing it to determine which factors best distinguish between one outcome and another. A knowledge of the items which predicted certain outcomes in the past can then be used to estimate how other people, embarking upon the same activity, are likely to behave. Such methods have been widely used in the field of criminology[1] and predictions of personal adjustment have been made in several other spheres as well; for example, in forecasting marriage adjustment, vocational aptitude, educational success, reaction to service life and battle conditions as well as children's response to care.[2]

A predictive approach in social research offers a means of summarizing a large amount of past experience in a systematic fashion, so that forecasts of the future can be made from it.[3] In general it takes the final form of a prediction table. The Mannheim and Wilkins study of the outcome of Borstal training[4] is an example of research which provided just such a table. From the past experience of boys passing through the Borstal system they wished to predict which were likely to benefit from it and which

---

[1] See for example, Mrs E. T. Glueck 'Predicting Juvenile Delinquency'. *British Journal of Delinquency*, Vol. 2, No. 4, April 1952, p. 279. The history of criminological prediction has been comprehensively reviewed in H. Mannheim and L. T. Wilkins' *Prediction Methods in Relation to Borstal Training*, H.M.S.O. 1954. It has also been discussed in Barbara Wootton's *Social Science and Social Pathology*, Allen and Unwin, 1959.

[2] See *The Rehabilitation of Children*, Edith M. H. Baylor and Elio D. Monachesi, Harper, New York, 1939. See also Monachesi's 'An Evaluation of Recent Major Efforts at Prediction', *American Journal of Sociology*, Vol. VI, 1941, p. 478.

[3] See particularly for a full discussion, L. T. Wilkins 'Some Developments in Prediction Methodology in Applied Social Research', *British Journal of Sociology*, Vol. VI, No. 4, December 1955, pp. 348–63. In the second part of this article (p. 354) he puts the essentials of the theory thus: 'In prediction we seek an equation which states that I may estimate the probability of success (or any other criterion) by considering other items of information, and giving them certain weight. Using the letter "X" to denote information and the suffix x_1 . . . to denote the particular piece of information, and the letter a, b, c . . . to denote the weight to be given, we might write ax, to mean the weight to be given, say, to the fact that a lad had previously been convicted a given number of times. Then we may write the generalized prediction equation: $ax_1 + bx_2 + cx_3 . . . = X$, where "X" is what we wish to predict. Of course in practice these equations do not predict "X" exactly but are the "best" estimators of "X" using the information put in, that is. $x_1 x_2 x_3 . . .$ The weights a, b, c, . . . are those which produce the best estimate of "X" within the limits of the input information'.

[4] H. Mannheim and L. T. Wilkins' *Prediction Methods in relation to Borstal Training*. H.M.S.O. 1954.

not. Benefit (or success) was seen as remaining free of conviction for 3½ years after discharge; failure as recidivism. Such predictions, the authors felt, would be of value to courts in determining the most appropriate sentence for young offenders. They drew up a table which enabled an estimate to be made of the chances of a boy succeeding or failing in Borstal training.

The factors in this prediction table (shown below) were those best distinguishing success from failure and each has an attached weight (or score) to indicate its relative importance in the set.[1]

For every factor which applies, count the number shown against the item: add together—the result is the basic score.

Factor	Add
If evidence of drunkenness	24·0
If any prior offence resulted in a fine	9·0
If any prior offence resulted in committal to prison or approved school	8·0
If any prior offence resulted in a term of probation	4·0
If *not* living with a parent or parents	7·5
If home is in an industrial area	8·0
If the longest in any one job was:	
Less than one month	11·7
Over 4 weeks up to 6 weeks	10·4
Over 6 weeks up to 8 weeks	9·1
Over 2 months up to 3 months	7·8
Over 3 months up to 4 months	6·5
Over 4 months up to 6 months	5·2
Over 6 months up to 9 months	3·9
Over 9 months up to 12 months	2·6
Over 12 months up to 18 months	1·3
Over 18 months	0

When the basic score is found it gives, by reference to a further table (over), the chance of success (or failure) of a particular boy.

[1]Ibid., pp. 145 and 146.

Group	Score	% Successful
A	0– 9·9	87
B	10–14·9	67
X	15–24·9	60
C	25–39·9	34
D	40 and over	13

If then a boy falls into the score group A it can be concluded, from the knowledge of how other boys had fared who scored similarly, that he has an 87 per cent chance of success. If, on the other hand he falls into group D only a 13 per cent chance of success can be expected.

That social work cannot be 'mechanized' is a truism which is sometimes used to discredit such statistical approaches to decision-making in this field. It is not suggested, however, that predictive devices should or could replace the personal judgement of the worker intimately concerned with a particular case. The claim is not that social work can be 'mechanized' but that it is possible to use certain 'tools' which can be provided by statistical methods. A prediction table can be one such 'tool'. There are at least three possible functions which it can perform in the casework field.

The accuracy of all decision rests upon the amount of relevant experience and information which the forecaster possesses. In some instances it does not matter very much if our forecasts are inaccurate, but in others it is essential that the margin of error should be kept to a minimum. Social workers are constantly having to make vital decisions which affect the lives of other people. Consequently it is clear that in social work decision-making any contribution to the 'storehouse of experience' upon which a caseworker can draw should be welcomed.

In the contemporary social work setting, however, the information which an individual can call on to help him make an accurate decision is primarily of an untested and personal nature. Little opportunity occurs during the pressure of day-to-day work to refer back to similar cases in the past or to check on the effect which certain factors or incidents had upon subsequent development. Further, it is difficult to judge the uniqueness of one's personal experiences or those of colleagues: and teaching lays only the foundation upon which experience must build. Nevertheless the potential 'storehouse of experience' which is available in social work is enormous; the difficulty is one of making it readily available to all those who wish to use it to supplement or compare their own range of experience. In child placement, Baylor and Monachesi suggested, 'the problems cannot be solved—in fact in many instances cannot even be recognized—without research that aims at making readily available the experience of the past'.[1]

This is a function which statistical enquiries and particularly predictive studies can perform. They can present the combined experience of many workers with many cases in a condensed and tested form. What casework methods of decision-making lack in the range of past experience that they can consider, statistical studies can provide: and the intensive knowledge of a case and the awareness of its particularly individual features which statistical methods are ill-fitted to deal with is amply provided by casework methods. Thus one of the contributions which a predictive study can make to casework practice is the provision of information, tested for its relevance, and based upon numerous cases.

A second function which these predictive techniques can fulfil in the partnership with casework springs from the first. They provide the caseworker with a yardstick against which to measure her own 'mental equations'. This is emphasized by Meyer, Jones, and Borgatta in their prediction study of whether unmarried mothers would relinquish their babies for adoption.[2] They concluded that the presentation of their findings did not imply that an empirical prediction could be substituted for the clinical judgement of the caseworker. 'It is the worker', they said, 'who still must decide, for each case, what the likelihood is that a girl will surrender or keep her baby, how appropriate the decision would be under all circumstances, how to handle the client's feelings and attitudes about the decision, and what service and treatment plans should be carried out. It does, however, challenge the worker to formulate more deliberately the basis for diagnosis and for planning, particularly in cases where the judgement and

---

[1] Ibid., pp. 494–5.
[2] Meyer H. J., Jones W., and Borgatta E. F. 'The Decision of Unmarried Mothers to keep or Surrender their Babies.' *Social Work*, Vol. 1, No. 2, April, 1956.

plan are at odds with the statistical probabilities of the case.'[1]

The third function which the prediction table can perform is to indicate where the limited amount of time and resources for intensive casework might most profitably be directed. If a child is boarded-out where the risk of failure is predicted as considerable the caseworker will clearly be forewarned that much supportive supervision may be needed and can plan accordingly. If the probabilities indicated by the table do in fact have this effect— of directing casework effort where it is most needed—the result might well be that the prediction table is 'disproved', in as much as its employment becomes in itself a new variable in the whole boarding-out situation, and one which obviously could not have been considered in the original study.

Thus in this study of foster care the choice of a predictive approach seemed particularly relevant to practical child care. From the research point of view it meant that a group of placements had to be selected where the outcome had been established. They then needed to be analysed to see whether there were any factors or groups of factors repeatedly associated with success or with failure. These results could then be used to construct a prediction table which would offer the information in an ordered and easily digestible form.

II

LIMITING CONSIDERATIONS

However, apart from these broad considerations of method, certain other factors also played a part in shaping the research. First, only 'pre-placing' data were collected and studied in terms of eventual outcome. Decisions about placements can only take into account and weigh up those items of information which are available at the time; many others are unknown, including all those which will subsequently be revealed during the placement. There is little to be gained therefore in demonstrating the predictive value of certain factors which would be, at least at the time, unknown to those responsible for deciding whether or not to make a particular placement; for instance, subsequent births and deaths in the foster family, illnesses or periods in hospital.

[1] Ibid., p. 106.

However, it might with some justification be argued that although the future incidents in a placement are unknown there are certain things which can be 'controlled'. For example, it could be suggested that through the work of a skilled caseworker a children's department does exercise a great deal of control and is able to introduce an influential variable into the whole situation. If a predictive study ignored this its results might be called into question. However, it is important to ask whether in practice the casework help offered to the child and his foster family can be regarded as different from one placement to the next in the way that sex or age might be. This does not seem to be the case. With the large turnover of staff and the increasing similarity in training the contribution which will be made by the child care officer can be, and normally is, regarded as a constant factor in all placements. This is not to say that it is unimportant in affecting success and failure, but that in deciding whether to go ahead with a placement it must be considered as potentially equal for each case, in the long-run at least. Since in a prediction study it is the differential effect of certain factors which is the important consideration, it becomes clear why the supervision factor is not included. When it becomes possible to claim that one placement is receiving significantly better or worse casework help than another then this factor needs to be included in a study such as this.

In this type of enquiry, then, 'post-placement' information, except about ultimate success or failure, is not essential. The aim is to 'recreate' the situation in which the person making the decision finds himself, with the same limitations on what is and can be known. Consequently, although it would certainly have been interesting to have gathered data from many placements as they progressed and were supervised, only the 'pre-placement' information and the final assessment have been used in this study.

The research was also limited to those placements which were of a long-term nature.[1] It was felt that long-and short-term placements exhibited rather different characteristics and raised somewhat different problems. Clearly both need to be studied, in the first place to determine whether the assumption of difference is in fact valid, but there are problems of dealing with them

[1] A more precise definition is offered in appendix II.

together which, because of its scale, this study was unable to overcome.

Another restriction was that only recorded material about the placements was used as the basic information. This meant using the case records of the child concerned and those of the foster parents. There were several reasons for this. In the first place it appeared reasonable that before searching for and tabulating new and as yet unrecorded information about the foster home placements an attempt should be made to utilize the material (in the form of case records) which was already available.[1] Further, the the study had necessarily to be retrospective.[2] In consequence collecting data over and above that already recorded would not have been easy. Since the placements to be studied had occurred some time in the past, information which might have been gathered from sources other than records (for example, by interviews with the officers concerned, with foster parents, with the staff of children's homes, and so on) would not have been equally available for all cases. Additionally a great deal of time would have been taken up in contacting and interviewing the numerous people involved in any one placement. Lastly, using case records as basic source material is less disruptive of the work of a children's department—no small matter—than lengthy discussions with child care officers or visits to foster homes.

There are at least two main disadvantages in relying upon recorded material. It is unlikely that the more intangible aspects of a case, known to the individuals concerned, can be taken into account although they may well affect success or failure. To this drawback must be added the fact that any errors or omissions in the recording are reflected in the results. Consequently these can be no better than the records which provided the basic information.

---

[1] It is interesting in this respect to read the remarks made by Erwin D. J. Bross in his book *Design for Decision*. (Macmillan New York, 1953). He says, for instance, 'in hospital administration . . . the day to day running of a hospital requires a tremendous number of records—case histories, accounting records, and so forth. Often this information is either thrown away, or, what is much the same thing, stored in ways which make the recovering of information a difficult, expensive, and time-consuming process. A hospital administrator who is faced with an immediate decision may feel that he does not have the relevant data which he needs, even though somewhere in the stacks of files in the basement there may be a ton of relevant files'. (pp. 258–9).

[2] This study could have taken the form of a follow-up enquiry but this approach had to be ruled out because of the time needed and limited resources.

Hence, the source material for this study was restricted to recorded pre-placement information about long-term foster homes and the knowledge of their ultimate success or failure.

III

THE SAMPLE OF PLACEMENTS

Deferring for a moment the discussion of what exactly is meant by the success or failure of a placement, the broad basis upon which the sample of placements was drawn will be described. It was necessary that the placements in the sample should have established their success or failure by the time they were assessed. Obviously this was not possible in any absolute sense but if a fairly long period from the date of placement was allowed to elapse before they were evaluated it seemed probable that most would be properly classed as either successes or failures. Eventually a group of placements was chosen which were made in the years 1952 and 1953 and the length of time before classification was fixed at five years exactly from the date of boarding-out. Thus those placements made in 1952 were assessed in 1957 and those made in 1953 in 1958.

From the little evidence available—for instance the study made by Trasler in Devon[1]—it would seem that in five or six years the majority of placements which are going to fail will have done so; but not all, of course. The Social Survey report on 'Children in Care and the Recruitment of Foster Parents' also provides some information on this point. This enquiry found that the average duration of all placements which were terminated for reasons other than discharge from care was $17\frac{1}{2}$ months.[2]

There were, however, three other conditions for the inclusion of a placement in the sample. First, only placements involving children who had been continuously in care during the five year period were included. To establish their success the placements had to run a full five years. Long-term cases which were apparently successful but discharged from care before the five years were up

[1] G. B. Trasler *In Place of Parents*. Routledge & Kegan Paul, 1959. This enquiry gave the information that of the unsuccessful placements which were considered, about 89 per cent had established their failure within a period of five years. (Table 16, p. 216.)
[2] P. G. Gray & Elizabeth A. Parr. S.S. 249, November, 1957, p. 28.

could not be included: had they in fact been exposed to the full risk period they might have become failures. In consequence those who failed in their foster homes before being discharged during the five years were also excluded: if they had not been, a disproportionate emphasis would have been placed upon the failures.

Second, to enable each placement to have an equal risk period of five years, only those involving children boarded-out on or before their thirteenth birthday were included. Since children go out of care on their eighteenth birthday, a child placed between 13 and 18 would not have been in care at the end of the five-year period. This particular limitation has both advantages and disadvantages. The main disadvantage is that some foster homes where older children were placed were excluded, thus underemphasizing to some extent the adolescent aspects of the problem. On the other hand when a child leaves school at 15 and starts work many of the placements made at this time or after are more like lodgings than foster homes. Thus even without the requirement of the thirteenth birthday bar it would probably have been necessary to omit many placements of children over 15 as not being 'true placements'.[1]

Additionally certain 'types' of placements were excluded. These were primarily the ones arranged privately, usually between the parent and foster parent, and those in which the foster parents were close relatives of the child.[2]

IV

THE DEFINITION OF SUCCESS AND FAILURE

Having briefly shown how the sample was defined it is now important to discuss what is meant by success or failure in a foster home, and describe the basis upon which the evaluations after the five-year period were made. There are many ways of deciding whether a foster home is a success or not. It is a relative concept, and varies from child to child. However, it is possible to employ some general definition which, although not being com-

---

[1] For example, 'Children placed in lodgings or in a hostel . . . or in residential employment are not boarded-out and so cannot be made subject to supervision under these regulations'. *Memorandum on the Boarding-out of Children Regulations.* Home Office 1955, para. 20 p. 4;.
[2] Other more detailed conditions are discussed in appendix II.

pletely accurate in assessing each case, classifies the majority correctly.

It was decided that it would be too difficult to group placements according to their degree of failure or success. A simple criterion was therefore sought which would distinguish the two outcomes. Briefly this was as follows: if, during the period of five years the child remained permanently in the foster home, then that placement was classed as a success: if he or she was removed then it was classed as a failure. The question immediately arises: are all permanencies to be considered successes and all removals failures? The short answer to the first question is yes. The second is more difficult. It would be misleading to classify all removals as failures; for example, a child may unavoidably have to be removed because of the death or long-term illness of the foster parents. However, if such cases cannot be considered failures neither can they with any justification be clearly reckoned as successes. For these reasons they were placed in an 'impossible to class' group which was completely excluded from the sample.[1]

A few removals were difficult to assess, but if there was any doubt the criterion resorted to was: 'are the circumstances leading up to the removal such that they might have caused the foster parents' own child to be cared for on a long-term basis by someone else?' If the answer to this was yes then the placement was put into the 'impossible to class' group and excluded. If the answer was no then it was retained and classed as a failure. This is perhaps a wider interpretation of failure than some would be willing to accept. The justification rests on the belief that to a child such removals were probably 'felt' to be failures or breakdowns and also that foster parents often seemed to give persuasive rationalizations in asking for a child's removal. They appeared to make a break when circumstances offered an opportunity; this possibly made it easier for them as well as for the child. It was particularly noticeable how often permanent removal was requested when the foster mother spent a short period in hospital; when she suffered the briefest of illnesses; when the family moved house or the child took up residential employment. However, this discussion of whether all removals were considered failures tends to obscure

[1] See appendix II.

the fact that the great majority seem to have been precipitated by failures in relationship.

This general definition of success and failure is admittedly arbitrary. However, it has the advantage of clarity and simplicity and is comparable from case to case. It has the drawback of not distinguishing some of the subtler forms of failure and success of which child care workers are aware. For instance, children may remain in a foster home for long periods where the placement is not entirely satisfactory or not meeting the child's needs as adequately as might be wished. There are others where the child is removed but where nevertheless, he derived something of value; partially succeeded, or had been more successful than with any other type of available provision. In this sense the definition of success and failure may be rather too rigorous, ignoring as it does the important administrative question of lack of alternative care.

The criterion employed in this study does not therefore establish the degree of failure or success. It might have been possible to have achieved this by using a more subjective definition; for example, if child care officers had been asked to assess on a scale various placements with which they were familiar. However, different people use different standards in making assessments and it becomes difficult to be sure that what one means by 'fairly successful' for instance, is the same as another's use of the term. As Trasler has pointed out: 'there is no accepted standard by which success in placement may be measured. The only indication of the degree of success that is achieved by boarding-out officers is to be found in the proportion of placements which are terminated by the removal of the child, because his relationship with the foster family has broken down. These are the cases which are indisputably breakdowns. . . .[1] Similarly Isobel Mordy claims that 'to a large extent the test of a failure of a placement in a foster home is whether the child has to be removed or not; although failures may be attributed to many causes'.[2] In *Accord*, the journal of the Association of Child Care Officers, it has been suggested that the most acceptable definition of breakdown is the 'permanent removal of a

[1] Ibid., p. 3.
[2] Isobel Mordy, *The Child Needs a Home*. Harrap 1956, p. 122.

child from a foster home in which he was placed either before or during his school life, if the decision to remove him is taken sooner than was originally planned and the fundamental cause is a failure of relationship within the home'.[1]

V

EXTRACTION OF DATA

Having identified the sample of placements and divided it into successes and failures the next problem was to decide which items from the information available in the case records of the child and the foster parent were to be noted.

As it was considered undesirable to load the study with preconceived notions about what was relevant information and what was not, all items available in more than 75 per cent[2] of the files were used. Thus, however important a piece of information might seem, if it was not fairly regularly available it remained unrecorded and unused. To do otherwise would have resulted in tabulations with large 'no information' categories and the statistical analysis of such material would have been unreliable. Some examples of facts which did not appear in many records were the child's I.Q.; early feeding history; psychiatric assessments, and so on. Consequently only those factors were included which would probably appear in a minimum of three quarters of the case papers.

This yielded 83 items of information about the child and 33 about the foster parents which were recorded on two check sheets. These sheets, when completed, contained all the information which was generally available in the records, in a standardized form. From them, it was possible to tabulate the results which are described and discussed in the following two chapters.

---

[1] *Accord*, Spring 1956, 'Suggestions for Research' (Anon.), p. 16.
[2] An initial pilot study of case records was made to establish the frequency with which data appeared.

3

DESCRIPTION OF RESULTS: THE CHILDREN

I

INTRODUCTION

IT should be clear that the primary concern of this study was not simply to describe successful and unsuccessful placements in terms of various factors but to identify those factors which together best distinguished one outcome from the other. The analysis which enabled this to be done and a prediction table drawn up is discussed in chapter 5. In this chapter and the next however, a straightforward description of the results most likely to be of general interest has been provided.

The discussion relies upon a fairly plentiful use of tables. In most cases tests of significance have been applied to them. The results of such tests are given below the appropriate tables as a measure of the probability that the variation between the successes and the failures is accounted for by chance. Results were considered to be significant only when the probability of this was 0·05 or less. That is, when only five times in a hundred might the distribution be expected merely through chance. Such tests provide the reader with an estimate of the confidence he can have that the results are in fact reflecting real differences.

One warning about the description which follows is perhaps warranted. It is important to remember that these results were achieved by studying placements of children who *were* boarded-out by a local authority. This certainly meant that the children's department had made various assumptions about which children were suitable for fostering, and by the same token, which foster parents were suitable. Any such assumptions introduce a selective process into boarding-out. For example, if it is widely felt that it is inadvisable to board-out enuretic children, except in special circumstances, then studying a sample of foster children will only reveal what part enuresis played in that selected group. Nothing will be known about the role it might have played had this policy or assumption not operated. If various authorities make dissimilar assumptions about such things, studies like this may not be entirely comparable from one area to another. If on the other hand, similar assumptions are made, the value of local studies is enhanced.[1]

II

SUCCESS AND FAILURE

In this sample of 209 placements, defined in the way discussed in the previous chapter, the rate of success was 52 per cent. Unfortunately there is almost no comparative information available about the success and failure of long-term placements. A few estimates have been made. Trasler, for example, recognizing the inadequacy of the statistics, suggests that 'many child-placing agencies are understandably reluctant to publish what may appear to be an unflattering index of their competence. But after these and other difficulties have been taken into account, it seems likely that between a third and two fifths of all long-term placements are unsuccessful'.[2] The only other enquiries providing either estimates or measures of the rate of failure are American and these found from 25 per cent to 50 per cent of the placements to be unsuccessful.[3]

However, it is not only the rate of failure and success which is

---

[1] A memorandum drawn up by the County Councils Association, however, does not support this view. They suggest that 'it seems likely that very divergent views are held by different County Councils and their officers upon the types of children suitable for boarding-out.... Children who in one county would be readily boarded-out with foster parents might in another county be regarded as wholly unsuitable for such treatment....' (Supplementary Memorandum by the County Councils Association to 6th Report from the Select Committee on Estimates, 1951–2—Included as Annex 10 to this report, p. 148).

[2] G. B. Trasler *In Place of Parents*. Routledge and Kegan Paul, London, 1960, p. 2. This estimate seems to be based upon a review of the information available from the reports of various Children's Committees in different parts of the country. (See relevant appendix in his unpublished Ph.D. thesis *Foster Home Success and Failure*, London, 1955.)

[3] See for example, E. M. Baylor and E. D. Monachesi *Rehabilitation of Children*. Harper. New York, 1937; W. Healy and A. Bronner *Reconstructing Behaviour in Youth*, Judge Baker Foundation Publication No. 5, Knopf, New York 1927, and S. van Theis' *How Foster Children Turn Out*. A study made for the State Charities Association—No. 165, New York 1924.

important. The duration of the placements which ultimately fail
is also of considerable interest. In some cases where the known
risk of placement is high, or alternatives not available, 'how long'
it is likely to last may prove to be an important factor to be taken
into account in deciding whether to place a child or not. In this
study the classification into success or failure was made after five
years; thus the removals, which characterized the unsuccessful
placements, occurred at varying intervals throughout this period.
In fact, as can be seen from table 1, just over 70 per cent of the
failures had occurred within two years.

TABLE I

The duration of the unsuccessful placements

	No.	
Under 6 months	21	⎫
6 months, under 1 year	23	⎬ 71
1 year, under 2 years	27	⎭
2 years, under 3 years	9	⎫
3 years, under 4 years	10	⎬ 30
4 years, under 5 years	11	⎭
	101	

Trasler found a very similar pattern for the duration of the
unsuccessful placements he studied: 76 per cent of them failing
within two years of being made.[1]

III

INFORMATION ABOUT THE CHILDREN[2]

Sex. The sample of placements concerned 103 boys and 106

[1] Ibid., table 17, p. 217.
[2] Several other factors about the children were collected and tabulated but were neither
significant nor of sufficient general interest to be included; for example, the child's religion
(85 per cent were stated to be C. of E. and only 4 per cent R.C.s), and his nationality
and colour. This latter factor has, since the years of this enquiry, become more important
but in this sample there were only three coloured children. It is interesting to note that
in the Baylor and Monachesi study (pp. 77–89) the nationality of the child's father (i.e.
in which part of the world he was born) proved to be one of the most discriminative
factors of favourable or unfavourable response to foster care. It seems reasonable to assume
that in the USA—and possibly increasingly in this country—boarding-out may be further
complicated by certain cultural differences.

girls—49 per cent and 51 per cent respectively.[1] These proportions are of some interest in view of the fact that there were more boys than girls in care in Kent during the period under investigation[2]— approximately 55 per cent to 45 per cent. This underlines the fact that proportionately more girls than boys are boarded-out, which was, indeed, the national pattern demonstrated in the Social Survey enquiry. That study showed that at the end of 1956, in the sample of children in care, only 37 per cent of the boys were boarded-out against 53 per cent of the girls.[3] However, although girls in care seem to have a better chance of being boarded-out than boys, there is no indication that placements with girls are any more successful.

Legal status. It would have been useful to have differentiated between 'types' of illegitimacy.[4] For example to distinguish the child of an unmarried girl, the child of a permanent union, or the illegitimate child of a married woman.[5] These are often very dissimilar situations and it is possible that illegitimacy does not have the same implications in each case. However, such an analysis did not prove possible; neither did a study of whether the child was aware of his illegitimacy, which in light of the conclusions of some investigators, might have been useful. Baylor and Monachesi, for instance, pointed out that '45 per cent of the illegitimate children who knew of their illegitimacy responded unfavourably to (foster) care, whereas this response was found in 28 per cent of illegitimate children without this knowledge'.[6] However, simply analysing success and failure by whether or not the child was legitimate did not show that one group was significantly more successful than the other, although there was a tendency for placements involving illegitimate children to be more successful. Trasler found a slight indication in the opposite direction.[7]

Children Act or fit person order. 39 per cent of the placements

[1] It will be remembered that five children were counted twice as they were boarded-out twice during the period 1952–3 and fulfilled the sample requirements on each occasion.
[2] This is also true for other periods in Kent.
[3] Ibid., pp. 13–14, tables 5a and 5b.
[4] For a useful bibliography on many aspects of illegitimacy see *Classified Bibliography on Illegitimacy*, National Council for the Unmarried Mother and her Child, 1958.
[5] See for example, Bowlby's discussion of 'types' of illegitimacy in his *Maternal Care and Mental Health*. W.H.O. Monograph No. 2, 1951. p. 93.
[6] Ibid., p. 157. See their table 77 on p. 156 as well.   [7] Ibid., p. 12.

involved children who had been committed to the care of the County Council on fit person orders. The average proportion of such children in care in Kent over the period of the study was 42 per cent. It is clear that this large percentage was not typical of the country as a whole.[1] The Social Survey, for instance, estimated that in March 1956 30 per cent of all children in care in England and Wales had been committed on orders;[2] for the same time in Kent the proportion was 46 per cent. It seems probable that wide differences like these reflect variations in court practices rather than local variation in the type of child coming before them. However there was no significant difference between the rate of success of placements with children committed to the County Council as a fit person, and those received through the provisions of the Children Act.

Age at placing. The likelihood of a successful placement being made decreased as the age of the child to be boarded-out increased. Table 2, however, shows that this pattern was not entirely regular. There was some indication that children placed between five and seven formed a group whose failure rate was higher than might have been suggested by the general trend. One possible explanation of this may be that schooling begins at five and the double stress of this and boarding-out proved too much for some children. However, as the totals in these groupings are rather small it is hazardous to draw any firm conclusions. Nevertheless there is no doubt that placements made with children from the younger age groups, particularly those under three, were the most successful. At the youngest end of the scale (under 1 year) the placement had about a 3 to 1 chance of success: at the other end (eleven and over) a 3 to 1 chance of failure. (See table 2.)

It is valuable to compare this result with other studies of a similar nature. Trasler, for instance, came to much the same conclusion. In his enquiry 69 per cent of the children placed under

---

[1] The Kent Children's Committee is very aware of this difference. In their report 1950–3 (p. 7) they say: 'In the light of experience gained some anxiety must be felt at the unusually large number of fit person cases which have been committed to care in Kent'.
[2] Ibid., p. 8.

TABLE 2

Child's age at placement

	Success		Failure	
	No.	%	No.	%
Under 1 yr.	13	77 ⎫	4	23 ⎫
1 under 2	21	62 ⎪	13	38 ⎪
2 under 3	15	65 ⎬64	8	35 ⎬36
3 under 4	14	56 ⎭	11	44 ⎭
4 under 5	8	50 ⎫	8	50 ⎫
5 under 7	12	34 ⎪	23	66 ⎪
7 under 9	13	52 ⎬41	12	48 ⎬59
9 under 11	8	47 ⎪	9	53 ⎪
11 and over	4	23 ⎭	13	77 ⎭
	108	52	101	48

(P is less than 0·01; d.f. = 1, table divided at 4 year level)
In this table and those which follow horizontal totals are omitted. Percentages add to a 100 across the table.

four were successful whereas for those of four and over the proportion was only 40 per cent.[1]

Theis, in a study undertaken in the 20s also had similar results. Although she used a criterion of success and failure rather different from that employed in this study, a fairly accurate comparison can be made with the information she gives about the number of foster homes each age group had experienced. Of those placed under five for instance, 81 per cent had no subsequent change of foster home, whereas of those placed over five only 48 per cent had no change.[2] She was also able to conclude that children placed under five made a much better adjustment in their adult life (her criterion of success) and that more than 90 per cent of them had found the foster relationship satisfactory in comparison with only 40 per cent of the older group.[3]

The information provided in the Healy and Bronner enquiry is limited by the fact that they dealt only with children over five. In spite of this they found that 'considering all types of cases and placings there is an advantage in accepting younger children for

[1] Ibid., p. 215.
[2] Ibid., p. 117.
[3] Ibid., p. 118.

placement. There appears to be a falling off of success with advancing years'.[1]

Although the Social Survey report made no specific attempt to classify placements as successful or unsuccessful an analysis was made of the age when a child was placed and whether the placement had terminated (other than by the child going out of care) for all children still in care at the end of 1956. It was found that a considerably greater proportion of placements made with children under the age of two years were 'still continuing' than those involving children more than two years old.[2]

In the Baylor and Monachesi study figures are given showing the response of children placed at different ages. No great difference was found in the groups placed under the age of eight but from this age onwards there was a decline in the rate of favourable response. 'The factor of age', these writers suggested, 'seems to play an important part in the entire foster home process; and in general it may be said that the older the child is before coming to the attention of the (placing) agencies the more difficult his adjustment becomes'.[3]

Studies such as these unanimously substantiate the results of our enquiry. The broad pattern which emerges is of a diminishing chance of successful foster care as the age of the child increases. This should not, however, lead automatically to the view that foster care should never be used for older children. It may be, for instance, that older children would have 'failed' just as frequently in other forms of care. In this sense boarding-out may still be the best alternative in spite of the apparently high risk of breakdown.

Behaviour problems.[4] The description and identification of behaviour problems from recorded material is fraught with difficulties. This is partly due to the fact that certain problems are more likely to be noted than others. Thus aggressive behaviour

---

[1] Ibid., p. 249.
[2] Ibid. See table 19 on p. 26.
[3] Ibid., p. 141. See also table 69, p. 149.
[4] These were considered to include: 'pronounced aggressiveness; unusual hot temper; repeated temper tantrums; frequent truancy; wandering; unusual destructiveness; acute sucking habits (not appropriate to age); pronounced sulking; sullenness; habitual pilfering; frequent rages; head banging; violent and repeated crying; recurrent nightmares; assertive enuresis; encopresis; pronounced sexual difficulties; excessive withdrawal; timidity; and delinquency,' each of which was mentioned specifically in the case records.

may attract more attention than excessive withdrawal or timidity. These possibilities must be borne in mind, especially as some writers have considered that it is particularly behaviour of an aggressive nature which gives rise to difficulties in the foster home.[1]

The results, as might be expected, show (table 3) that placements with children exhibiting behaviour problems were significantly more likely to fail than those placements involving children without such difficulties.

TABLE 3

Behaviour problems exhibited before placement

	Success		Failure	
	No.	%	*No.*	%
Behaviour problems	14	30	32	70
None recorded	94	58	69	42
	108	52	101	48

(P is less than 0·01)

Enuresis was considered separately, since it seems to have been thought of as one of the more common adverse factors in the fostering situation. The problems of the enuretic were particularly high-lighted during the widespread billeting which resulted from wartime evacuation. Titmuss devotes some attention to it in his *Problems of Social Policy*. He quotes a leader from the *Lancet* of October 1939: 'Somewhat unexpectedly', remarked the writer, 'enuresis has proved to be one of the major menaces to the comfortable disposition of evacuated urban children . . . every morning every window is filled with bedding, hung out to air in the sunshine. The scene is cheerful but the householder depressed'.[2] Although almost 25 per cent of the placements with children of three or more involved enuretics the results in this study do not support the conclusion that evidence of enuresis before placement can usefully distinguish between those likely to be successful and those not. Admittedly of course pre-placing

[1] e.g. in Susan Isaacs' *The Cambridge Evacuation Survey*, p. 93 et seq., and the study of Goldfarb (W. Goldfarb 'Infant Rearing and Problem Behaviour'. *American Journal of Orthopsychiatry*. Vol. XIII No. 2, April 1943, p. 249).
[2] R. M. Titmuss *Problems of Social Policy*, H.M.S.O., p. 721 et seq.

information does not show whether enuresis cleared up after placement or whether it started in those not previously affected, and it is always difficult to judge at what age a child can be considered enuretic.[1]

Medical record. In many case the medical history was very sketchy; in others, particularly those who had been in a children's home or nursery, it was adequate. The information was thus extremely uneven both in quantity and quality. However it was possible to use certain specific items of medical information. For instance, the handicaps from which children might be suffering when boarded-out can be roughly divided into 'mental' and 'physical'. Those with a physical handicap were involved in only eleven placements (about 5 per cent)—and seven of these succeeded. Though of course these numbers are too small to be reliable it is nevertheless of interest to see that they do bear out the information given in the Social Survey report. This pointed out 'that a gratifyingly high proportion, 62 per cent, of placements made with children with handicaps . . . are successful, perhaps because extra care is taken in selecting the foster parents for those children who require special care'.[2]

In contrast to this they found that only 30 per cent of those children with mental disabilities (educationally sub-normal;

TABLE 4

Mental disability[3] established before placement

	Success		Failure	
	No.	%	No.	%
Mental disability	6	29	15	71
None recorded	102	54	86	46
	108	52	101	48

(P lies between 0·05 and 0·02)

[1] Arbitrarily no child under 3 was considered enuretic. Another difficulty was to distinguish those children who were only nocturnal enuretics. Since information was not always precise about this no attempt was made to treat it separately.

[2] Ibid., p. 29.

[3] The mentally 'disabled' included those adjudged maladjusted; mentally ill; mentally defective; those authoritatively classified as severely retarded, and the educationally subnormal. (As a result of the 1959 Mental Health Act some of the terminology and classification has been changed.)

mentally defective, and maladjusted) were succeeding.[1] Although once more the numbers involved are rather small it can be seen from table 4 that our results substantiate this finding—with a rate of success for a similar mentally handicapped group of only 29 per cent.

IV

THE CHILD'S EXPERIENCE OF CARE

Institutional[2] *experience before placement.* From the results of many studies of the effect of institutional care upon the social and psychological development of children[3] it might reasonably be expected that the children who had spent some time in residential care before being placed in foster homes would be less successful than those who had not. Goldfarb was, in fact, able to demonstrate an association between the amount of institutional care in infancy and the subsequent failure of foster care,[4] and Trasler also found this to be the case. Of course, as he points out, such results need to be treated cautiously for some children might have spent 'a longer-than-average period in institutions because they were suffering from emotional disturbances which later caused the failure of attempts to board them out'.[5]

In view of this evidence the institutional history of the children in the placements was studied in some detail. In the first instance this was done irrespective of when residential care had actually occurred. For example, a simple count was made of all the institutions the children had been in before placement (table 5). This showed that although the differences were not statistically significant there was a trend in the expected direction: those placements where the child had been in an institution were rather less successful than those where they had not. However, the actual number of institutions did not differentiate in any way between subsequent success and failure.

[1] Ibid., p. 29.
[2] The terms 'institutional' and 'residential' have been used interchangeably.
[3] See in particular, of course, J. Bowlby, *Maternal Care & Mental Health.* W.H.O. monograph series, No. 2, 1951.
[4] See William Goldfarb. 'Infant Rearing as a Factor in Foster Home Placement'. *American Journal of Orthopsychiatry,* Vol. XIV, No. 1, January 1944, p. 162.
[5] Ibid., pp. 210 and 211.

TABLE 5

The number of institutions in which the child had lived

	Success		Failure	
	No.	%	No.	%
None	20	63	12	37
One	52	49	53	51
Two	17	53	15	47
Three or more	19	48	21	52
	108	**52**	**101**	**48**

(P lies between 0·20 and 0·10; d.f. = 1, table divided
none/some)

When the history of the children involved in the placements
was analysed in terms of the amount of time they had spent in
institutions interesting and significant differences did appear
(table 6). Somewhat surprisingly, the placements with children
who had been in institutional care for more than one year but less
than two were more successful than those with children who had
only experienced this form of care for less than a year and just as
successful as those with children who had had no such experience.
However, the highest rate of failure (74 per cent) was found in
those placements with children who had spent three years or
more in institutions.

TABLE 6

Total time the child had spent in institutions

	Success		Failure	
	No.	%	No.	%
None	20	63	12	37
Under 1 year	45	51	43	49
1 under 2 yrs.	29	63	17	37
2 under 3 yrs.	7	44	9	56
3 yrs. or more	7	26	20	74
	108	**52**	**101**	**48**

(P is less than 0·01; d.f. = 2; table divided none/
under 2/2 or more)

A more specific analysis was made of the effect of institutional experience in infancy upon foster home success. It might have been expected, for instance, that those children who had been in institutional care sometime in their first two years of life would prove less successful when boarded-out. This was not so. Table 7 in fact shows a tendency in the opposite direction, although the difference is not statistically significant.

TABLE 7

Whether the child had been in an institution during his first two years of life

	Success		Failure	
	No.	%	No.	%
In an institution	55	57	42	43
Not in an institution	53	47	59	53
	108	52	101	48

(P lies between 0·20 and 0·10)

This lack of significance might be partly accounted for by the fact that many of the children who had not been in institutions would not have been in care in their first two years; and it was established during the study that the later a child came into care the significantly less successful he was likely to be in a foster home.[1] In general, of course, it has to be pointed out that many of the studies, such as those quoted by Bowlby, which showed the ill-effects of institutionalization upon young children relied for comparison upon children in 'families', in their own homes, or in foster care. It is by no means certain that children who are destined for long-term care experience anything comparable with these fairly normal situations as alternatives to residential care in early life. Consequently in table 7 and those which follow in this section, it should be remembered that largely unknown alternatives are being compared with institutional care.

Although whether or not a child had been in an institution

---

[1] Placements with children received into care before they were one year old had a 63 per cent rate of success: those with children who were seven or more when taken into care only 37 per cent.

during his first two years of life[1] did not discriminate between the successes and the failures it was thought that the duration of such care during that period might be more significant. This proved to be the case as can be seen from table 8. The placements with children who had spent less than a year in institutional care in their first two years of life, were more successful than those with children who had stayed longer than a year. Surprisingly, this group was also more successful than the placements with children who had never been in an institution at all.

TABLE 8

Length of time child spent in institutional care
in his first two years of life

	Success		Failure	
	No.	%	No.	%
None	53	47	59	53
Under 1 year	43	64	24	36
1 year or more	12	40	18	60
	108	52	101	48

(P lies between 0·02 and 0·01; d.f. = 2)

If, instead of the first two years of a child's life, the period considered is extended to the first five, the result is still not significant when a simple distinction between 'had' or 'had not' been in institutional care is made, but the tendency remains for those who had been in some such care during this period to be the more successful group. However, when this information is presented in terms of the total time spent in institutions in the first five years a pattern very similar to that in table 8 once more emerges (table 9). Placements with children who had been in residential care more than two years during their first five years were a particularly unsuccessful group: and again, those placements with children who had spent some time, but less than two years in institutions were the most successful. Children who had never been in institutions in their first five years do not stand out as either particularly successful or unsuccessful.

[1] If, instead of 'institutional care during the first two years of life', only the first year is considered a similar result is obtained.

TABLE 9

Time spent in institutional care during the first five years

	Success		Failure	
	No.	%	No.	%
None	31	45	38	55
Under two years	68	61	44	39
Two years or more	9	32	19	68
	108	52	101	48

(P lies between 0·02 and 0·01; d.f. = 2)

Making a somewhat similar analysis, Trasler could not substantiate the hypotheses that failure in foster placement was associated with spending at least two years of the first five in residential care, or at least half of the first three. However he considered that since children who were over five years of age when received into care would rarely have been in institutional care in their early years, an older and hence less successful group of children would be found in the 'no institutional care' category. With this in mind he tabulated data on the total time spent in institutional care in the first years of life for that group only which was received into care under the age of five. A very significant distribution emerged from this which supported his hypothesis as well as the contention that the factor of age had been obscuring the pattern in the original analysis when all the children were considered irrespective of their age at admission to care. His analysis is given in table 10 in a slightly amended form.[1]

TABLE 10

Time spent in institutional care during their first three years of life by children under five when received into care—Trasler

	Success		Failure	
	No.	%	No.	%
None	20	91	2	9
Less than 1½ years	15	68	7	32
1½ years or more	24	44	30	56
	59	60	39	40

[1] Ibid., p. 210.

If our data are similarly tabulated for the group of placements involving only children received into care under five, the results are less conclusive and the pattern significantly different (table 11). Those who had not been in institutional care at all in their early years still do not appear the highly successful group that Trasler found, whereas those cared for residentially in their first three years for periods of less than 18 months appear just as successful. However in both studies those children who had spent more than eighteen months in institutional care in their first three years were singularly unsuccessful.

TABLE 11

Time spent in institutional care during their first three years of life by children under five when received into care

	Success		Failure	
	No.	%	No.	%
None	26	59	18	41
Less than 1½ years	54	62	33	38
1½ years or more	8	32	17	68
	88	56	68	44

(P lies between 0·05 and 0·02; d.f. = 2)

In pursuing Trasler's line of thought, a study of the effect of institutional care on the success of a group of placements where the children were of a limited age range suggested itself. For this purpose all those placements made with children under the age of four were selected and success and failure analysed by their institutional experience. No significant difference appeared whichever way this relationship was examined.

From these various ways of analysing and tabulating the relationship between institutional care before placement and subsequent success or failure in foster homes certain conclusions can be suggested and hypotheses constructed. Generally it would appear that it is not so much the number of institutions a child has passed through which is prejudicial to subsequent placement but the amount of time involved. The longer this experience lasted the more adverse the effect seemed to be on subsequent fostering.

However, perhaps the most important result was that children who had spent relatively short periods in institutions sometime before placement were likely to be as successful, if not more so, than those who had had no institutional experience. This seemed particularly true of periods spent in institutional care in infancy.

This might suggest that the value of the limited period in a home or nursery prior to boarding-out ought to be reconsidered. It may be that this provides a useful stable transitional environment for the child recently accepted into care; or, through having had the child in residential care for a reasonable period of time (a) the children's department is better armed with relevant information about that child, and (b) in cases where the child is placed from the home or nursery no immediate pressure is applied on the field staff to make quick decisions—as when the child is moved from one foster home to another or placed directly upon reception into care.

These results may also suggest that the function of the reception centre in pre-placement assessment could be strengthened. In fact in this study only 17 per cent of the children involved had at any time passed through a reception centre and only 4 per cent had on this occasion been boarded-out directly from such a centre.[1] Neither group was any more successful than those who had not been in a reception centre but since this form of provision was limited it seemed likely that the children selected to go there were the more disturbed and possibly poorer risks in placement.

Clearly these results do not entirely match-up with Gordon Trasler's nor do they substantially support other studies,[2] although they do not contradict them. The main difference is that studies such as Goldfarb's and Lowry's found children who had not been in institutions at all more successful in foster homes than those who had.[3] · [4] However, Goldfarb for instance,

---

[1] Pioneer work in reception centres was carried out in Kent, at New House, Merstham. This experiment has been described in Hilda Lewis' book *Deprived Children*, O.U.P., 1954. When this centre was closed the Kent Children's Committee opened a similar establishment elsewhere.

[2] e.g. I. Mordy, *The Child Needs a Home*, Harrap, 1956, Appendix, pp. 122–3.

[3] Ibid.

[4] L. G. Lowry, 'Personality Distortions in Early Institutional Care' *American Journal of Orthopsychiatry*, Vol. X, 1940, p. 567.

compared a group without institutional experience with another which had been in residential homes throughout the *whole* of their first three years of life. Periods of institutional care less than three years were not considered. If the same procedure had been used in this study similar results to his would have been obtained; indeed there seems unanimity that long periods (two years or more) of institutional care in infancy are associated with later foster home failure. Previous investigations however, seem to have paid little attention to the effects of relatively short periods in institutions. More enquiries are obviously needed of the effects of these shorter spells of residential care upon children of different ages.

Previous experience of fostering.[1] Some 43 per cent of the placements involved children who had already had experience of foster care. It is perhaps unexpected to find that those children who had been fostered once already were more successful than those who had never before been boarded-out (table 12).

TABLE 12

The number of times the child had been previously fostered[2]

	Success		Failure	
	No.	%	No.	%
Never before	55	46	65	54
Once	42	64	24	36
Twice or more	11	48	12	52
	108	52	101	48

(P lies between 0·05 and 0·02; d.f. = 1; table divided fostered/not fostered)

[1] In this section 'foster home' includes any foster home irrespective of whether it had been selected or supervised by the Children's Department. For example, Child (Life) Protection homes. These are privately arranged between parent and foster parent and supervised under Child Protection Regulations when they are reported, but in many cases the foster mothers fail to inform the welfare authority that they are receiving a child for payment. Further, if a child had been living with close relatives (e.g. an aunt or grandmother) this was not considered to be a foster home.

[2] In this table there were 18 placements in which the child had previously experienced *only* a private foster home (12 of these were successful).

In view of this result it seemed important to establish whether the children who had already been in a foster home had been successful or not. The same criterion for success and failure could not be used as in the general sample; first because all these placements had terminated, and second because they included all 'types' of placements (short-term and private, for instance). For this reason a different twofold classification of previous placements was used: 'had failed in a previous foster home' (a removal because of a breakdown in personal relationships), and 'had not experienced a definite failure'. The latter group is not necessarily to be considered 'successful'—it includes terminations which were unavoidable, short-term placements, and those where the child was returned to his parents. The results of this analysis are given in table 13.

TABLE 13

Child's previous experience of foster care (where this could be judged)

	Success		Failure	
	No.	%	No.	%
None	55	46	65	54
Failed at least once	28	52	26	48
No definite failure	21	72	8	27
	104	51	99	49

It seems from this that the large proportion of successful placements made with children who had been previously fostered could in part be accounted for by the 'quality' or 'lack of failure' in those placements. It may be that it is having a 'good experience' of previous fostering that prepares the child well for subsequent boarding-out. Or again, there may be a selective process opearting which only gave the opportunity of a second placement to those who seemed to stand a very good chance of success. Children whose difficulties in a foster home become apparent in the first placement may not in fact be tried again.

Second placements thus appear to be fairly successful. It is interesting to speculate whether, like many other things, successful adjustment in a foster home is something which has to be learned. Likewise it would be interesting to know whether the additional information gained about a child from his reaction to foster care led to more appropriate future placement decisions. In line with these results it was found that the children who had previously been fostered for longer periods were rather more successful than those fostered for a shorter time.

The number of moves the child had experienced. An analysis was made of the number of moves the children in these placements had experienced whilst in care (holidays and short periods in hospital being disregarded). From the results presented in table 14 no support can be obtained for the often assumed relationship between a large number of previous moves and failure in the fostering situation.[1]

TABLE 14
The number of moves the child experienced whilst in care

This placement was:	Success		Failure	
	No.	%	No.	%
Direct	16	57	12	43
First move	52	52	48	48
Second move	10	36	18	64
Third move	14	56	11	44
Fourth or more	16	57	12	43
	108	52	101	48

Placement preparation. Throughout child care literature 'preparation' for boarding-out is continually stressed. For example, Jean Charnley states that 'the keynote of success in all child placement is careful preparation'.[2] However it was difficult to estimate from the records how much preparatory contact the

---

[1] A study was undertaken by the Kent Children's Department of a group of 888 children who had been in care on January 1, 1952 and were still in care on December 31, 1956 to discover how many moves (excluding placements in reception centres and holidays) they had experienced during this period. The average number of moves for the children in this study was 1·24, and 38 per cent of them were not moved at all. ('Report of the Children's Committee 1953–58' K.C.C., p. 18).

[2] *The Art of Child Placement*, Minneapolis, 1955, University of Minnesota, p. 3.

worker had had with the child or indeed with the foster parents. Nevertheless it was thought that the number of recorded contacts the child had had with the foster parents before placement would provide an approximate indication of the extent of preparation. Naturally those children who had been in the home previously or who were there already (i.e. those received into care from a private foster home but continuing to be boarded-out there) had the best preparation in terms of contact with the foster parents. The results showed very similar rates of success for all the placements where there had been less than five initial contacts and those without any preparatory visits did not stand out as particularly unsuccessful. Although not significantly so, those with five or more contacts and those already in the home were a rather more successful group.

V

THE CHILD'S FAMILY

Information regarding many of the aspects of a child's family background was not available, or only available in a few cases. Trasler found a similar situation in his study. 'The most serious deficiency', he claimed, 'in our case material, proved to be an almost total lack of information about those aspects of his family history which might be significant to the child's heredity.'[1] However, several factors for which information was generally available were tabulated in this study.

Age at separation from mother.[2] The child's age at permanent separation from the mother is not necessarily identical to his age at last reception into care. In fact 38 per cent of the placements in the sample were made with children who had been received into care on the last occasion from outside their immediate family group: they were, in fact, no longer in the daily care of either parent. From table 15 it can be seen that there is a significant continuous decline in the rate of successful fostering with increasing age at separation from the mother. Some have assumed

---

[1] Ibid., p. 208.
[2] Information was collected about age of separation from father and similar results obtained. There was some difficulty of course as many children were illegitimate.

that children who have been deprived of maternal care early in life are more likely to have difficulty in forming satisfactory relations with foster parents than those who make the break at an older age. In fact the opposite seems to be the case. The children who experienced their mother's care for some years appeared to settle less easily in a foster home.

TABLE 15

Child's age at permanent separation from his mother

	Success		Failure	
	No.	%	No.	%
Under 1 year	48	63	28	37
1 under 3	31	53	27	47
Over 3 years	29	39	46	61
	108	52	101	48

(P is less than 0·01; d.f. = 2)

Trasler obtained somewhat different (although not significant) results in his study.[1] If his table in respect to the child's age at separation from his mother is condensed (table 16) it can be easily compared with table 15.

TABLE 16

Child's age at separation from mother—Trasler

	Success		Failure	
	No.	%	No.	%
Under 3	49	54	42	46
3 and over	32	68	15	32
	81	59	57	41

However, most other studies support our conclusions. For instance, although Baylor and Monachesi did not provide directly comparable results they did study the child's age at 'leaving home'. Their conclusions have some relevance. 'For the sake of argument', they suggested, 'it may be said that if a break is to occur, it had better take place when the child is young, for the effect of

[1] Ibid., p. 209.

having to leave home when one's orientation has been established may easily result in a disaster or at least in a long period of mal-adjustment. This statement', they concluded, 'is supported by the data presented. . . .'[1]

Our results may also fit in with those of other investigators who have stressed the importance of a child's attitude to, and his awareness of separation from his family. For example, Adah Baxter in a small-scale study suggested 'that foster home place-ment ultimately failed for the child whose attitudes seemed to imply that she did not want and could not accept separation from her own family'.[2] If this conclusion is valid it would seem reasonable that not wanting, or not accepting separation from his or her family may be related to the child's awareness of his 'own family'. Such awareness is likely to be less vivid among children separated from their parents very early in life. In this respect Miss Dyson's comment is of interest. 'It is thought,' she notes, 'that older children who have lost happy homes through sickness or death settle more easily in homes than foster homes.'[3] 'Happy homes' is, of course, a weighty qualification.

Children whose mothers were dead. Although only 14 per cent of the total sample involved the placement of children whose mothers were known to be dead, the results were highly signi-ficant. It appeared quite clear that the loss of a mother was associated with failure in a foster home (table 17).

TABLE 17

Children whose mothers were dead

	Success		Failure	
	No.	%	No.	%
Mother dead	7	24	22*	76
Mother alive	101	56	79	44
	108	52	101	48

(P is less than 0·01. * Includes six orphans)

---

[1] Ibid., pp. 163 and 164.
[2] 'The Adjustment of Children to Foster Homes' in *Smiths College Studies in Social Work*, Vol. VII, No. 3, 1937, p. 191.
[3] D. M. Dyson *The Foster Home and the Boarded-Out Child*, Allen & Unwin, 1947, p. 46.

It was established that the mother being dead was also significantly associated with both the child being over four at placement and being over three at permanent separation from his mother. Consequently it would seem that in those cases where the mother was dead the child had often experienced some mothering and possibly a fairly normal home life. The fact that many placements with such children failed lends support to the suggestions of both Baxter and Dyson. It is also interesting to find that Baylor and Monachesi discovered that those children whose mothers were dead had a significantly higher failure rate than those whose mothers were living—either at home or elsewhere.[1] The social and psychological problems of fostering bereaved children would seem to call for further study.

The home background. It was extremely difficult to establish the child's background in any precise fashion. Only two indices were in fact employed: first, whether the child's parents were living together normally at the time of placement and second, whether the NSPCC had ever visited the home before the child was taken into care. The first index did not differentiate in any way between the successes and the failures although it is perhaps interesting to note that 20 per cent of the parents were living together, in the sense of not being separated or divorced, at the time their child was placed.

The selection of the second index—NSPCC visits—was suggested by Donnison's study of the neglected child. In his enquiry into the services offered such children and their families before they were received into care he used seven indices as a 'measure' of neglect. One of these was 'whether an NSPCC inspector had visited a family and decided there was sufficient danger of neglect to justify the formal opening of a case and the regular visits which that involves'.[2] In using all his indicators he found that the families known to the Society 'were much worse neglected than the rest'.[3] However, this factor did not discriminate between the successes and failures in this study although in as many as

[1] Ibid, see table 17, p. 96.
[2] *The Neglected Child & the Social Services*, Manchester University Press, 1954, p.26.
[3] Ibid., p. 80.

52 per cent of the placements the child's family was known to have been visited by the NSPCC before he was taken into care.[1]

There were few other items of information which might have provided guides to the quality of home environment from which the children had come: added to which there was very little generally recorded data about the parents themselves. Little or nothing was recorded about the father in 66 per cent of the cases and in 34 per cent information about the mother was similarly lacking.

Child's siblings. Most of the children placed came from what might be regarded as 'large' families. 28 per cent had at least four siblings: a further 14 per cent three, and 22 per cent two brothers or sisters. Thus some two thirds came from families with at least three children. Only 15 per cent were 'only' children—most of them illegitimate. In 69 per cent of the placements in the study the child had a sibling or siblings who were also in care. A problem which looms large for any children's department is the extent to which the separation of such children is or is not justified. Table 18 sets out the various groupings and re-groupings of siblings which occurred at the time of the placement. Only those placements involving children with all or some siblings also in care are considered. The results are not significant and there is no clear evidence that placements which necessitated a child being separated from brothers or sisters were more likely to fail than any other. There was in fact a slight tendency for those separated from siblings both before and after placement to be the most successful group.

TABLE 18
Changes in sibling groupings

	Success		Failure	
	No.	%	No.	%
Placements in which the child:				
remained separated from his siblings	35	56	27	44
was separated from them	11	44	14	56
was kept with all or some of them	21	43	28	57
was reunited with them	5	—	3	—
	72	50	72	50

[1] In his sample Donnison found 43 per cent—see his p. 79.

The whole problem of how best to provide for a family of several children in care serves to illustrate some of the difficulties faced by child care officers. For instance, although in general it seems desirable that siblings should not be separated this will probably reduce their chance of being boarded-out. Taken in conjunction with the evidence of table 18 (that the success of a placement seems unaffected by whether or not siblings are placed together) this might well suggest that an undue, and possibly unjustifiable emphasis is being placed upon keeping brothers and sisters together. As in so many other decisions in child care however several different and often competing objectives have to be taken into account. For example, by splitting up the children of a family its eventual reunification may be jeopardized, or children already deprived of parental care may be further deprived of the support of their brothers and sisters. To reiterate the qualifications of the last chaper: there is no one exclusive criterion of a successful placement against which all decisions can be tidily measured.

These then are some of the more interesting items of information which emerged from an examination of the records about the children who were boarded-out. The discussion has enabled certain other studies to be considered and a number of wider questions to be raised. Some of these will be explored further in the final chapter. A study of boarding-out must, of course, also take into account information concerning the foster parents. This is discussed in the next chapter.

4

DESCRIPTION OF RESULTS:
THE FOSTER HOME

I

OTHER CHILDREN IN THE FOSTER HOME

IT was found that the rate of success was highest (75 per cent) where there were no other children at all in the foster home and lowest (29 per cent) where there were four or more. However, it is an over-simplification to talk of other children in the foster home without distinguishing their different status. In fact they can be clearly divided into three groups: the children who were offspring of the foster parents; siblings of the child placed; and other non-related foster children.[1]

The number of the foster parents' own children living in the foster home is given in table 19. The result is significant and shows a considerable difference between placements where there were no 'own children' and those where there were. The most successful placements were made in foster homes where the foster parents either had no children of their own or had none at home under the age of eighteen.

If instead of looking at the number of 'own children' at home at the time of the placement, the ages of these children are considered, some very significant results are obtained. There is a particularly low rate of success where there is any child of the foster parents under five. The rate improves steadily as the ages

---

[1] Throughout this chapter 'child' means anyone under the age of eighteen. 'Other' children in the foster home means children in the same household, forming part of the foster family unit. There was only one case in which a child could not be placed into one or other of these categories—this occurred when the foster mother had charge of a grandson. He was treated as an 'own' child. 'Own children' included those adopted.

TABLE 19

The number of foster parents' children living at home

	Success		Failure	
	No.	%	No.	%
None	56	65	30	35
One	34	44	44	56
Two	14	42	19	58
Three or more	4	33	8	67
	108	52	101	48

(P is less than 0·01; d.f. = 1; table divided none/some)

of the 'own' children at home increase, but at no age does it become nearly so high as when there is no child at all. A table showing the number of 'own children' under five is presented below.

TABLE 20

The number of foster parents' children under five

	Success		Failure	
	No.	%	No.	%
None	96	59	68	41
One	11 }	27	28 }	73
Two	1 }		5 }	
	108	52	101	48

(P is less than 0·001; d.f. = 1)

An even more significant result was obtained when the age relationship between the foster child and the foster parents' own children was examined. The presence of a son or daughter of the foster parents whose age was within five years of the foster child's was clearly a prejudicial factor in the placement situation. Where there were two or more such 'own' children the rate of failure was higher still. The marked difference between the failure of placements where there were 'own' children within five years of the foster child and the success of those where there were not is clearly shown in table 21.

TABLE 21

The number of foster parents' own children within five years of the age of the placed child.

	Success		Failure	
	No.	%	No.	%
None	75	68	36	32
One	28	37	47	63
Two or more	5	22	18	78
	108	52	101	48

(P is less than 0·001; d.f. = 1; table divided none/some)

From these results it seems clear that there is an association between failure and the presence of offspring of the foster parents in the home. This is particularly accentuated when an 'own child' is under five years of age or is less than five years older or younger than the foster child. The sex of the children involved does not appear to influence these general conclusions.

In a little over a quarter of the placements a child was boarded-out in the same foster home as brothers or sisters. However, unlike the presence of offspring of the foster parents, this in no way differentiated between the successes and the failures—in spite of the fact that in most cases at least one of them was no more than five years older or younger than the child in the sample. The only qualification to this general conclusion might be that where the child was placed with two or more siblings—rather than with just one or on his own—the possibility of failure seemed slightly greater. Some children were also placed in foster homes in which there were other foster children neither related to them nor to the foster parents. Again this did not appear to affect the outcome one way or another. Thus it seems clear that failure is not associated with the presence of *any* other child or children in the foster home but specifically with the foster parents *own* children—particularly young ones and those near the age of the placed child.

[1] It was not possible to determine exactly whether the age difference was more or less than five years in a few cases. When this occurred, for example if the age of the placed child was three and that of the foster parents' own child eight, and no dates of birth were available, it was considered that the children were within five years of each other's age.

Evidence drawn from other studies tends to support these findings. Trasler obtained similar results although his conclusion distinguished between various sex groupings. 'Of those children', he wrote, 'who were placed in a home in which the foster parents' own child was of the same age and sex, no less than 87 per cent ended in failure; while no such difference appears in those placements in which the foster parents' own child was of the other sex, or was more than three years older or younger.'[1] Mulock Houwer found the most successful placements to be those where 'a difference of four years or more (in either direction) existed between the foster child and the foster parents' own child of the same sex'.[2] Bowlby suggested that placing a foster child of the same age and sex as the foster parents' child gave rise to friction and was a situation to be avoided whenever possible. He pointed out that in such circumstances the foster child is 'thought of too much for his uses as a playmate and too little for himself. Moreover,' he contended, 'situations of jealousy and rivalry are apt more often not to arise when age or sex are different.'[3] Drawing on her own experience Jean Charnley wrote, 'I have learned to shy away from placing small children in foster homes with own children of similar ages and sexes. The inevitable rivalries are too threatening for the foster child and the disappointment to the own child in the unsatisfactory companionship can be too severe.'[4]

These conclusions differ from those of this study only in that they consider placements where 'own children' are of the same sex as the placed child to be more unsuccessful than those where they are not of the same sex. However, a small scale study undertaken as long ago as 1932 came to exactly the same conclusions as this enquiry. 'The ages of children', it reported, 'actually living in the homes at the time they were first used are significant because these were the children with whom the foster child was expected to assume a sibling relationship. The figures show that in those homes which we are calling successful the sons and daughters were largely adolescent or adult. This seems to show',

[1] Ibid., p. 223.
[2] Quoted by Bowlby as a verbal communication. Ibid., p. 127.
[3] Ibid., p. 127.
[4] Ibid., pp. 177 and 178.

the writer continued, 'that successful foster homes rarely contain "own children" near the age of the foster children'.[1]

It is worth recording the opinion of Burlingham and Freud on this question of foster-sibling relationships. They emphasized that the problem of jealousy and competititon between brothers and sisters was presented in evacuation in the new form of jealousy between foster brothers and sisters. 'Children never feel friendly,' they pointed out, 'towards a new born addition to their family. They sometimes pretend to do so; at other times they are mollified by the smallness and complete helplessness of the newcomer. The newly billeted foster brother on the other hand, is very often neither small nor helpless. He usurps rights which the other child is unwilling to give up. The billeted newcomer for his part is deeply conscious of his second-rate position and is embittered by it.'[2]

II

THE FOSTER PARENTS

Social class. A person's occupation is usually taken as an index of his social status or class. The Registrar-General in his Census reports uses a fivefold classification of occupational groups to estimate social class.[3] This classification was applied to the foster fathers in our sample but no significant difference appeared between their success as foster parents. Trasler using the same classification likewise found no variation.[4] However, the Registrar-General's fivefold classification has certain limitations. One drawback is that the middle group (social class III—skilled workers) tends to have a very wide 'spread'. For example, in this study it included the somewhat different occupations of railway shunter and senior salesman in a large store. Consequently, and since it also contained over half the foster fathers in the sample,

---

[1] Virginia Dudley, 'Foster Mothers: Successful and Unsuccessful', in *Smiths College Studies in Social Work*, Vol. 3, No. 2, December 1932, pp. 156–7.
[2] Dorothy Burlingham and Anna Freud, *Annual Report of a Residential War Nursery*, 1942, p. 30.
[3] The five groups which are distinguished are: professional; intermediate; skilled; partly-skilled, and unskilled. For a more detailed breakdown of occupations see the Registrar-General's *Classification of Occupations*.
[4] Ibid., p. 218.

it seemed worth trying to split it by employing some different system of classification.

A method was used, therefore, which offered four classifications rather than five. Primarily this contracted the two sets of extreme groups in the Registrar-General's system and expanded the centre group into two divisions (table 22). Into group A were placed the professional people, those with independent means, large farmers and so on. Group B comprised those broadly identified as 'white collar workers'. These included bank clerks, supervisors, shop owners, commercial travellers, salesmen, smallholders, and such like. Those in Group C were distinguished from Group B by being manual rather than 'white collar' workers. They included the craftsmen and tradesmen (e.g. bricklayers, printers, toolmakers, potters, blacksmiths, carpenters, etc.). The new class D is mainly composed of the Registrar-General's semi-skilled and unskilled workers: for example, bus conductors, semi-skilled factory workers, and labourers. This classification is to some extent arbitrary and imprecise; however, its main function was to split the Registrar-General's group III classification. In some cases no information was available about occupation and these have been excluded.[1]

TABLE 22

A fourfold classification of social class of foster parents based on the foster father's occupation

Social class group	Success No.	%	Failure No.	%
A	6	40	9	60
B	11	30	26	70
C	27	53	24	47
D	50	57	38	43
	94	49	97	51

(P lies between 0·05 and 0·02; d.f. = 3)

As it stands this distribution is statistically significant but be-

[1] Those excluded were cases where there was no foster father (12); where he was retired and his previous occupation was not stated, and where the job was too vaguely described for classification. Altogether 18 placements were excluded for these reasons.

cause the placements where the social class of the foster parents could not be accurately assessed were concentrated in the successful group (14 out of 18) the results should be treated cautiously. It would appear, however, that the lower the socio-economic class of the foster parents the more successful a placement is likely to be. Further investigation of the influence of class values and expectations upon the outcome of placements with children of different ages and from different social backgrounds would seem to be warranted.

It is of further interest to compare the percentages of foster parents in each class group (according to the Registrar-General's system) with the figures given in the 1951 Census Report for Kent.[2] This gives the social class distribution of occupied and retired males aged 15 and over. Since it would be very unlikely that foster fathers would be selected who were under 21 or over retiring age distortions at both ends of the age scale may occur, and it is impossible to make a correction for this. However, the breakdown by class of the foster fathers involved in the placements and the Kent population as a whole is nevertheless of some interest and is given in table 23 (those whose occupations could not be ascertained again being excluded).

TABLE 23

Comparison of the socio-economic class of foster fathers in the sample with the distribution in the county as a whole

Class (Registrar-General)	Sample 1952–3 %	Kent 1951 %
I	2·1	4·6
II	14·7	16·5
III	58·6	52·3
IV	14·7	14·2
V	9·9	12·4
	100·0	100·0

This result is similar to that obtained in the Social Survey

[1] General Register Office. *Census 1951 of England and Wales*, H.M.S.O. County Report—Kent, p. xiix, Table T.

enquiry in which the authors concluded that 'there are fewer foster mothers in the extreme income groups than would be expected having regard to their age distribution. The highest income group is appreciably under-represented among the foster mothers.'[1]

Age of the foster mother. Although this factor is not significant the distribution in table 24 does show a tendency for the older foster mothers to have provided the more successful placements. Those under forty seem less successful as a group than the over-forties while the under 30s stand out as the least successful. However, it was established that there is a highly significant relationship between the foster mother being over forty and there being no 'own children' under five or five years older or younger than the placed child. It could, therefore, be the important relation-ship between these factors and success and failure which is being reflected. However, against this it was also found that there was a significant relationship between foster children being over four at placement and the foster mother being over forty. Clearly the older foster mothers are getting the older children, wno as a group are less successful than the younger.

TABLE 24
The age of the foster mother[2]

	Success		Failure	
	No.	%	No.	%
21–30	14	42	19	58
31–40	39	48	42	52
41–50	40	58	29	42
51 and over	15	58	11	42
	108	52	101	48

(P lies between 0·10 and 0·05; d.f. = 1; data grouped 21/40 and 41 and over)

Other studies have also found a rise in the rate of success with the increasing age of the foster mother. Trasler claimed that

---

[1] Ibid., p. 36.
[2] The ages of the foster fathers were also considered but it was found that the pattern followed very closely the distribution in table 24 and they have not been tabulated.

'the large proportion (about 67 per cent) of failures among placements with foster mothers under the age of forty is most striking'.[1]
Baylor and Monachesi concluded that in their investigations
'generally speaking . . . the data indicate that better results are
obtained with the older foster mothers and fathers'.[2] For example,
they found that in '73 per cent of the times that children were
placed with foster mothers over 35 years of age a favourable
response to care resulted, as against 56 per cent for those in which
the foster mothers were 35 years of age or less'.[3]

From the Census Report for Kent it is possible to get an
estimate of the proportion of women who might be available as
foster mothers in each age group. Married women in the age range
20–69 were taken from the Census to make a comparison with
the age distribution found in this sample of placements.[4] Necessarily the comparison is approximate but it does indicate that the
31–40 age group is particularly over-represented in the study, and
that the two older groups are under-represented. The distributions
in table 25 may well be the result of a definite policy of avoiding
the older women as foster mothers for long-term placements, or
a difference in willingness to act as foster mothers.

TABLE 25

*Comparison of age groupings in the sample of foster
mothers with overall age distribution for Kent*

| | Sample | | | Kent Census |
	No.	%		%
21–30	33	16	20–29	18
31–40	81	40	30–39	25
41–50	69	34	40–49	26
51–60	16	8	50–59	19
61 and over	10	2	60–69	12
	209	100		100

Foster parents' previous experience. No difference existed between the relative success of those placements where the foster

[1] Ibid., p. 219.
[2] Ibid., p. 320.
[3] Ibid., p. 323.
[4] *Census 1951.* County Report—Kent, p. xlii, Table P.

parents had had foster children before and those where they had not. There are, however, two other aspects of this factor which must be considered: the number of foster children the foster parents had previously had and how long they had cared for them. The first of these did not show any significant relationship to the success or failure of the placement. There was, however, a fairly strong tendency (not quite statistically significant) for those who had already looked after foster children for more than a year to be associated with successful placements more often than those who were acting as foster parents for the first time or who had previously only looked after a foster child for less than a year. What is of particular interest in table 26 is that placements with foster mothers who had never had a foster child before were more successful than those with women who had been foster mothers for periods under a year. Presumably the foster mothers in this latter group of placements will have had mainly one or two short-stay cases before this placement. This suggests that selecting long-term foster mothers on the basis of their performance as short-term foster mothers may not be a reliable procedure.

TABLE 26

Length of time foster mothers had previously acted in that capacity

	Success		Failure	
	No.	%	No.	%
Never	54	53	48	47
Under 1 year	26	40	39	60
1 year—under 4 years	15	65	8	35
4 years and over	13	68	6	32
	108	52	101	48

(P lies between 0·01 and 0·05; d.f. = 1; table divided less than 1 year/1 year or more)

Childless foster parents.[1] For many reasons, but primarily

[1] Included as childless marriages were those in which all the children were dead or where there was only a child by a former marriage. However, in no case was there a step-child actually living in the foster home at the time of the placement. Although physically childless those foster parents who had adopted children were not classed as childless. There were eleven such cases, five of which succeeded.

because the obvious motive of childless couples in fostering is not always considered 'ideal', some doubt is often expressed about the wisdom of using such foster homes. As Trasler pointed out, 'infertile couples in particular tend to approach foster parenthood as a substitute for physical parenthood, and may try hard to preserve the illusion that the child is their own, sometimes to the extent of denying his parentage and his previous experiences which they have not shared'.[1] There are clearly dangers in this sort of situation but the results in this study do not support the conclusion that placements with childless foster parents are unlikely to be successful. In fact the contrary appears to be the case, and Dyson's conclusion that 'childless couples often made excellent foster parents . . .'[2] would seem to be substantiated as can be seen from table 27.

TABLE 27
Childless foster parents

	Success		Failure	
	No.	%	*No.*	%
Childless	38	67	19	33
Not childless	70	46	82	54
	108	**52**	**101**	**48**

(P is less than 0·01)

This result is significant but clearly there is an overlap with the fact that there are no 'own' children in the homes of childless couples, and this factor has already been demonstrated as highly significant.

The lack of a foster father. The absence of a foster father in the home has often been considered an adverse factor. Consequently it is possible that only in exceptional cases were children boarded-out under such circumstances. The number of placements using foster homes without foster fathers was small (6 per cent) but there was no indication that they were less successful than the

[1] Ibid., p. 113.
[2] Ibid., p. 28.

C*

others.[1] Of twelve such placements nine were successful. Trasler similarly found that those foster homes without a foster father were slightly more successful, though not significantly so, than those with both husband and wife.[2]

Some of the factors which seem to distinguish most clearly between the successful placements and the unsuccessful appear to concern the structure of the foster family. In particular whether or not there are children of the foster parents seems a crucial consideration. Significant factors such as these, however, were further analysed to establish exactly which combination possessed the greatest power to predict the outcome of placements. This is discussed in the chapter which follows.

[1] Of the twelve placements made where there was only a foster mother, eight were with boys only and four with girls only. Of the former seven were successful, of the latter two. The twelve placements were further analysed by the status of the foster mother. In four cases they were single women (two successes); in five they were widows (all successful); and in three they were divorced or separated (two successful).

[2] Ibid., p. 220.

5

THE PREDICTION TABLE

I

THE STATISTICAL BACKGROUND

So far the results of this study have been described in terms of
the relationship of individual factors with the criterion—success
or failure. However, social behaviour is very complex and if the
relationship between each factor and success or failure is examined
as if it were independent of all others this complexity is ignored
and no really efficient prediction table could be developed. Many
factors related to success or failure in a foster home will in turn
be related to each other. For instance, although the death of the
child's mother seemed to have a prejudicial effect upon foster
home success, bereaved children were also older at placement and
this too was seen to be an unfavourable factor. Hence the importance of the one cannot be judged without considering its relationship with the other.

An analysis of such inter-relationships would be useful in itself,
but it is also an essential step in producing an efficient prediction
table. Efficiency requires the optimum use to be made of the
material available. This does not mean that a large number of
factors have to be included, for some of them are almost alternatives (for instance, 'age at separation from mother' and 'age at
admission into care'), whilst others overlap (for example, the
'age of the foster mother' and 'own children living at home'). If
all that was required was to show which factors were associated
with the outcomes in the sample studied this might not matter.
But a prediction table aims to forecast the likelihood of success
in those placements yet to be made. Under these circumstances

every factor included will introduce more error as well as more precision. The problem is to choose just that set which maximizes the accuracy: in other words to make such a selection that one more or one less item would reduce the table's predictive value. When such a set has been selected the table is as efficient as possible, given the range of information available.

Thus to make such an optimum choice it is necessary to identify overlap and duplication between the factors. To include an item largely accounted for by another which has already been chosen will almost certainly mean that the additional error outweighs the extra discrimination. The statistical process by which these inter-relationships were considered and the most efficient combination of factors selected is a form of multivariate analysis.

II

THE TABLE

A brief outline of the methods employed in this multivariate analysis is provided in appendix III. It is sufficient here to point out that the factors eventually identified as the most efficient for predicting success and failure are not all of equal importance. Hence the analysis also provides a measure of the weight to be attached to each. This has been incorporated as a 'score' for each item in the final table set out below.[1]

Prediction Table

If the following applies at placement add the appropriate score:

	Add
There is a child of the foster parents under five	33
The child's own mother is dead	28
The child is four or more years old	23
The child has exhibited behaviour problems	17
The child has *not* been previously fostered	15
There is a child of the foster parents whose age is within five years of that of the child to be placed	14

[1] In the table:
   (a) behaviour problems include those things listed on p. 46.
   (b) previous fostering includes placing by a local authority, voluntary society or private arrangement. Placements with immediate relatives (siblings, uncles or aunts or grandparents) are not counted.
   (c) adopted children are counted as 'own'.

As it stands this table only shows which are the most discriminatory factors and their relative importance. If applied to a particular case it gives a total score without indicating what that score means in terms of the probability of success or failure. The next step therefore, was to apply the table to the original sample. Having scored each placement, and knowing its outcome, a subsidiary table was built up which attached estimates of the probability of success or failure to the various scores.[1]

Distribution of scores

Score	Success No.	Success %	Failure No.	Failure %
I Under 15	16	94	1	6
II 15–29	47	80	12	20
III 30–49	23	51	22	49
IV 50–79	19	27	50	73
V 80 and over	3	16	16	84
	108	52	101	48

$$(r\emptyset = 0.52)$$

From this it can be seen that a placement scoring less than fifteen (i.e. in which none of the six adverse factors were present) indicated a 94 per cent chance of success. On the other hand, with a score of over 80 the rate of success could only be expected to be 16 per cent. Hence any long-term placement which is being contemplated can be scored from the knowledge of six factors and this can be translated into an estimate of its chance of being successful.

One word of warning is perhaps important. The set of factors must always be regarded as a whole. If one item is replaced or re-weighted the accuracy of the table is reduced. Each factor has been selected as an element in a combination. Thus these variables should not be thought of as separate causes. There may be some causal relationship between each and success and failure, but it

[1] The score intervals were selected to give approximately a 50:50 break in the middle group and not too few cases in the extreme groups.

would be incorrect to assume this directly from their inclusion in the table for, as it has already been stressed the influence of the selected factor takes into account and reflects other overlapping variables as well. In this sense each of those items selected might be regarded as the 'best representative' of a group of influences rather than being an independent 'cause' in itself.

It might also seem reasonable to expect the table to predict not only the final outcome but also the length of time those ultimately failing were likely to last. That is, the more favourable the score the longer the placement might be expected to continue before failing. However, this proved to be an untenable assumption. Clearly, the factors selected for the prediction table, although the best set for distinguishing between the failures and successes generally, did not provide any indication of the 'length of time before failure' amongst the failure group. If the point at which a placement is going to fail is to be predicted it would seem that a new set of factors would have to be selected.

III

VALIDATION

Until the prediction table has been applied to a different sample it cannot be considered validated. Ideally, such a check should be made on as large a scale as possible, but all that could be done within the scope of this enquiry was to apply it to a new sample consisting of all those long-term placements made in Kent during 1954. The same definition of the sample was used as for the main study and a record made in each case of only those six factors used in the prediction table. These were scored appropriately and the placements grouped in their respective risk categories. They were then assessed for success and failure after a five-year period and the outcomes checked with the prediction.

The validation sample consisted of 108 cases. The success rate was almost identical with that in the main study—51 per cent compared with 52 per cent. When these 108 placements had been scored for the six factors according to the prediction table the distribution of scores was as follows:

Distribution of scores in the validation study

Score	Success No.	Success %	Failure No.	Failure %
I Under 15	4	80	1	20
II 15–29	24	75	8	25
III 30–49	15	54	13	46
IV 50–79	10	30	23	70
V 80 and over	2	20	8	80
	55	51	53	49

$$(r\emptyset = 0.44)$$

Clearly the small size of this check sample has some drawbacks. The two extreme score groups (I and V) do not really provide enough cases to make a reasonable comparison with the results in the original study. The most favourable score group in particular is insufficiently represented. Consequently it seemed appropriate to combine groups I and II, and IV and V, and compare them with the same combined groups in the original sample.

Comparison of prediction scores in the original and validation studies

Score	Original Study: % Success	Validation Study: % Success
I and II: Under 30	83	76
III: 30–49:	51	54
IV and V: 50 and over	25	28
	52	51

It can be seen that there is some loss in discriminative power. The correlation coefficient is reduced from 0.52 to 0.44. Nevertheless the result is satisfactory and can be regarded as validating the prediction table. There are several possible reasons why the degree of accuracy has decreased. First, the sample is smaller. The most appropriate check would have been with a sample at least the size of the original study. However limited resources prevented this from being done. Second, the grouping of scores was to some extent arbitrary: there is no guarantee that the choice was the most appropriate from the point of view of ensuring the greatest precision when the table was generally applied.

Clearly it would be most interesting to make a number of further studies in Kent to see to what extent the prediction table retains its accuracy. In addition it might be applied and tested in other and contrasting areas. There are without doubt certain features of the work of the Kent Children's Department which are unrepresentative; one which has already been mentioned being the high proportion of fit person order cases in care at any one time. Any such subsequent enquiries could be carried out fairly quickly and would test the validity of the results to a greater extent than has been possible here. In general further validation studies, preferably on a larger scale, need to be undertaken before such a prediction table as this could be confidently employed in practice.

IV

SOME SECONDARY RESULTS OF THE ANALYISS

An integral part of the statistical analysis which produced the prediction table was an examination of the interrelationship of many factors with each other as well as to the criterion success or failure. Some of these interrelationships have already been mentioned in chapters 3 and 4. However, it is of interest to show more specifically the pattern of association between such things as age and mental disability or enuresis and sex. Clearly it is impossible, and not particularly useful, to comment on all these relationships and in the following discussion only those which were significant or seemed of general interest are included.[1]

There was, as might be expected, a close connection between those factors which broadly speaking give some indication of whether or not a child is 'disturbed'. Behaviour problems,[2] for instance, were significantly associated with both mental disabilities[3] and enuresis. They were also related to the child having been in institutional care for more than two years and to his age at placement. The older children exhibited behaviour problems significantly more often than the younger. It is of interest to see

[1] For further information see the matrix of concomitance in appendix IV.
[2] See p. 46.
[3] See p. 46.

that mental disability was related to the same set of factors, with the exception of enuresis—the mentally disabled were not significantly enuretic. The fact that a child's mother was dead was linked with enuresis, behaviour problems and mental disability and seems to be closely woven into what might be termed the 'adjustment' complex of factors. Likewise, as many commentators have pointed out,[1] long periods (over 2 years) in institutional care are associated with—though not necessarily causing—enuresis, behaviour problems and mental disability. As has already been emphasized, this may merely be a reflection of the tendency to keep the more disturbed children longer in residential care, rather than residential care producing these symptoms.

The factor of age is connected with most of these items and appears to be very much a crucial variable. For instance, those children who had a mental disability; suffered enuresis; showed behaviour disturbance, or had lost their mother through death, were more likely to be the older children.

There is another distinct interrelated group of factors again closely associated with age. For example, illegitimate children were younger than legitimate at placement; were likely to have been separated from their mothers when less than three years old; to have been previously fostered and to be in care under the provisions of the Children Act, 1948, rather than a fit person order.

Although there were fewer factors concerning the foster home, these were more tightly interrelated. The foster mothers over 40 were likely to have no children at home and to have acted as foster mother on one or more previous occasions. In contrast, childless couples had, significantly, not done the work before—suggesting perhaps that they were seeking a pseudo-adoptive situation by means of a 'once and for all' fostering.

If the factors primarily concerning the child and the factors mostly concerning the foster home are examined for their interrelationship it is possible to draw certain conclusions about placing policy as it actually occurred. To see, in effect, which sort of children were repeatedly placed in which sorts of homes. When this is done, perhaps the most surprising thing is that there are so few significant patterns. However, a number of general state-

[1] See pp. 47-54.

ments can justifiably be made from the analysis. Young children went to young foster mothers with pre-school children of their own. Older children went to older foster mothers without young children. Children with behaviour problems more often went to couples who had children of their own but where these were more than five years old, although still within five years of the foster child's age. Childless couples got children of all ages but significantly without behaviour problems. Children who were placed in a foster home with 'own' children of about the same age were more likely to be girls than boys; to have been more than 2 years in residential care beforehand and to have shown evidence of behaviour disturbance.

Looking at these reflections of placing policy which the multivariate analysis threw up one is struck by the levelling-out process which appears to be operating. In many instances, older foster mothers, who have been shown to be rather more successful, got the older children who were the greater risks. Young children who seemed most likely to settle comfortably and easily into a foster home went to the younger foster mother with her own young children—and this group was shown in the study to be particularly unsuccessful. It might be concluded that the children most likely to succeed go to the foster homes most likely to fail, and vice versa. There is possibly a balancing of 'resources' against 'problems'. On the other hand children with behaviour problems went to the homes where there were 'own' children of competing ages, and childless couples, whom the research showed to be a successful group, received the least disturbed children. The exceptions to this generalization thus seem to involve the disturbed child. He appeared to go to the homes least likely to succeed. Perhaps there was an element of Hobson's choice in this!

As well as showing something of the pattern of actual placing policy, whether conscious or not, this analysis suggests those factors which commonly influenced the decisions of child care officers: age of child; his degree of stability or disturbance, and perhaps sex on the one hand, and the age of the foster mother and other children in the foster home on the other. In contrast, the mentally disabled; the enuretic, and those fostered before, did not go significantly often to any particular type of foster home.

A more systematic approach to the study of actual placement policy along these lines would be of considerable interest and value. The brief discussion offered here is based upon material incidentally thrown up from the main stream of the enquiry. Hence this is by no means a comprehensive analysis of the inter-relationship between factors: it does, however, illustrate the problem of 'overlapping' discussed previously and begins to demonstrate the remarkable complexity of social phenomena—a complexity ignored at risk of misrepresentation and distortion.

6

DISCUSSION

I

THE PLACE OF RESEARCH IN CHILDCARE WORK

In many ways this study has over-simplified the problem of making 'best' decisions in child care, for it has focused upon but one of many possible forms of provision. The situation rarely arises in which the child care officer only faces the choice of whether or not to go ahead with a particular foster home placement. Normally such a decision is complicated by the need to take into account the effectiveness and availability of alternative courses of action. For instance, if suitable residential accommodation is available or there is a large number of potential foster homes to choose from, a placement about which there was some uncertainty would probably not be used. If, on the other hand, there were fewer acceptable alternatives sights might be lowered and the same foster home taken up. Decisions are always, one hopes, made in the interests of the child's welfare but they are also determined by the limitations imposed by the provisions available. The child care officer may, faced with the need to secure 'immediate care' for a child, be forced to choose between a restricted number of mediocre alternatives. Such unfortunate realities are largely ignored by this study.

However, although no apology is required for the failure of the enquiry to make a comprehensive analysis of decision-making in child care there remains the danger that because it deals with only one part of the problem it may inadvertently suggest that the accumulation of more information will guarantee improvements in boarding-out. This is only partially true, for it is just as essential to extend the scope, quality and availability of alternatives. If this were achieved fewer foster home placements might be made merely because nothing else was more suitable at the time. In other words it would become easier to decide not to board-out a child.

Similarly more knowledge about one possible decision may fail to do justice to other alternatives about which less is known. To safeguard against this many parallel studies of the relative success of other forms of care are urgently needed. It is also possible that more information may be of very limited practical value unless the means exist by which it can be utilized. The consultant psychiatrist, to offer a familiar example, may give the best possible advice about how a child's needs can most effectively be met but if the provision recommended is not available little is achieved. Or again, if it is demonstrated that a certain type of family is the most appropriate for certain foster children this is of little use unless such people can be recruited. Faced with dilemmas like these research may be dismissed as having no practical value: however it is often overlooked that its findings may play an important part in the argument for additional resources; an argument increasingly revolving around 'evidence'. If it can be shown that a certain form of provision is needed for certain children but is in short supply, this can be a persuasive weapon in the hands of committees or chief officers. In this sense the research itself may help to win the extra resources needed to absorb the new-found knowledge into day-to-day practice.

Indeed the problem of insufficient resources is a crucial part of our understanding of decision-making in child care. In fact, scarce resources, whether created by increasing demand or rising standards, are a significant part of the work of children's departments as of other social work organizations. In many cases it is quite impossible to defer or avoid making a decision and hence choices inevitably become circumscribed by the resources of the moment. The child destined for long-term care may be especially penalized by this situation, for instead of comprehensive plans being laid, a series of decisions may be taken, throughout a long period in care, each of which is influenced primarily by short-term current posibilities.

An important step in improving the standard of child care

work will be made when the urgency or 'immediacy' of decisions is reduced;[1] for decisions which have to be made at short notice with inadequate knowledge and with only a limited range of alternatives are unlikely to be as sound as ones made under less pressure. In an unhurried atmosphere more relevant information can be collected and it is possible to 'wait' for the most appropriate provision to become available. The development of preventive work and the earlier identification of children at risk may go a long way to achieving this and the present re-emphasis upon the reception centre as a means of both assessment and diagnosis could also play a part. It has been suggested elsewhere that one of the reasons why children who had been in residential care for a short period before boarding-out seemed a successful group was to be found in this freedom from the 'immediate' need to decide on a foster home, together with the accumulation of additional information. Broadly speaking relevant knowledge plus an unhurried atmosphere, plus a real choice of alternative forms of care are likely to add up to better decision-making. Prediction tables, however accurate they may be, are obviously only part of this general equation. But their important contribution is in providing measures of 'risk'. Different administrative situations will doubtless determine the levels of risk which can generally be accepted.

One of the urgent requirements in many fields of social work[2] is for more detailed case studies of how decisions are actually made—as opposed to how they are thought to be made: to know more precisely, for instance, what factors, pressures, or ideas and beliefs are actually taken into account in boarding-out a child and what weight is attached to the numerous different considerations. It is also important to be aware of the areas of ignorance which force us to make unfounded guesses or untested assumptions. One of the things which became evident during this study, for example, was the difficulty in determining just how long a child was likely to be staying in care. Hence many foster home placements which clearly began as short-term grew into long-

[1] For a description of child care work undertaken in the midst of 'urgency' and 'immediacy', see John Stroud's novel, *The Shorn Lamb*.
[2] A valuable recent contribution is Professor D. V. Donnison's *Social Policy and Administration* (National Institute for Social Work Training Series), Allen and Unwin, 1965.

term arrangements, often successfully but incidentally 'blocking' a number of foster parents who had been specifically chosen for short-term cases. A similar problem arises in the provision of short-stay residential care: where it is impossible to predict how long individuals are expected to remain the phenomenon of 'silting-up' or blocking may occur. A prediction study which aimed at forecasting how long children received into care were likely to stay would certainly make a valuable contribution to appropriate decision-making—both in regard to individual children and the use of resources. At the moment the conventional 'reasons for admission into care' are, one suspects, poor indicators of how long the child is likely to require care.

There are many other examples of the ignorance which surrounds the process of making decisions. For instance, from the material collected in this study it seemed common for the children most likely to fail to be placed with the foster parents most likely to succeed—and vice versa. If such choices are being made, to what extent is the staff aware of them? If they are, can this process be considered a justifiable policy? If we are to improve the quality of our decisions in child care not only do we need more time, resources and information we also need to know much more about how decisions are made. Case study methods in child care have made some contribution to our understanding, but they tend to emphasize some aspects of the situation and underplay others. Little is ever said, for example, about the influence of scarcity upon ultimate decisions. The concern to show people's reactions to situations and decisions often means that the analysis, in administrative terms, of how the situation arose and how and why the decisions were taken is overlooked. The more we learn about the process of decision-making the better will we be able to judge how improvements might be made.

Prediction tables like the one developed in this study begin to help. How far this approach can contribute to better decision-making will depend upon many of the factors already discussed. In addition, of course, it will depend upon the extent and accuracy of our records of past experience and the willingness of workers to use its findings. The stage has not yet been reached when these can confidently be recommended to them, more remains to be done. Nevertheless some attention can be paid *now* to such things as the standard of recording, the collection of material, the framing of hypotheses and questions, and the undertaking of further preliminary studies. Such work will lay a sound foundation for future enquiries, for research is essentially cumulative in character, ideally one study building upon another. However, in the final analysis research is only likely to flourish and be used in an atmosphere of irreverence towards accepted assumptions and current theory; criticism of what is being achieved, and an awareness of what is actually being done.

II

THE DEVELOPMENT OF GENERAL HYPOTHESES

It may be argued that although the study of a particular activity with a view to providing a prediction table helps us to make more accurate decisions it does not lead to a 'real' growth in knowledge. Knowledge, that is, of the essential nature of human behaviour and interaction. Of course, it must be readily admitted that this is not the main aim of a prediction study, but it must also be remembered that the pursuit of knowledge, unless this is regarded as an end in itself, is related to its value as a means of making reliable forecasts of future events. Why else should general laws be so eagerly sought? Nevertheless in taking the data of past experience and presenting them in an easily digestible form a prediction table can fulfil the important secondary function of suggesting the direction which subsequent investigations might take. This can be discussed in a number of ways: the construction of 'reasonable' hypotheses is one.

There are various patterns of possible general explanation into which the results of this study might be fitted. For instance, it might well be possible to explain the success of foster homes in terms of whether the foster mother was able to assume the role of a natural mother to the child and whether the child could assume the role of natural offspring. The problems and difficulties of normal parenthood are borne and overcome primarily because the children are 'yours': they are part of the parents and to reject them is in many ways to reject oneself. To bear the additional difficulties, tensions, and exasperations which foster children create one would seem to need this safeguard to an even greater extent. Likewise the child in the testing circumstances of a foster home may need to be able to feel an 'own' child if he is to cope with the many difficulties he faces over a long period. In the foster home with an own child both the foster parents and the foster child may be brought up against the reality of their true relationships and as a result find it difficult to assume the roles by which they can best overcome the daily crises. Similarly where the child comes into care at an older age or after a parent's death he may find it equally hard to take this role, especially when this can mean denying the reality of his own parents, of whom he may have vivid recollections. The visits of the child's parents to the foster home are often regarded as a 'disturbing influence', and this too may represent a situation in which the asusmption of a parental role by the foster parents is challenged and undermined.

It is interesting to analyse such a hypothesis against the historical background of boarding-out. Before the last war foster care, where it occurred, tended to be long-term and often grew into *de facto* adoption. The child frequently took the foster parents' name and such things were accepted as normal by many children's organizations. These foster parents clearly fulfilled a parental role, largely unchallenged by the child's own parents or by the possibility of his eventual removal. Reunification with his family was unlikely; the child was in care to receive its benefits and be sheltered from an undesirable environment. This situation, it might be argued, enabled foster parents to tolerate many of the difficulties common in boarding-out, since they could employ what might be termed the 'strategy of identification': that is, regarding the child as if it were really theirs. Now however, with the aim of rehabilitation and the general expansion of short-term care, children's departments are anxious that the subsequent reunification of the child with his family should not be prejudiced by allowing the placement to slip into semi-adoption. The roles of parents and foster parent become, at least in principle, differentiated. The visits of the child's parents, the possibility of removal, the insistence that the child uses his own surname and does not address his foster parents as mother and father, all make it clear to them that theirs is not the parental role. Hence they are inevitably discouraged from using the manoeuvre of identification by which they might have been able to deal with the problems which arise. At the same time, one suspects, they are left in considerable doubt as to the exact nature of the foster parent role.

If this hypothesis were substantiated by further investigation it might well become evident that some breakdowns, particularly in long-term placements, are associated with the fact that child care organizations, for what may be excellent reasons, ask unskilled and untrained foster parents to do a difficult job in what for them may be an unnaturally difficult way: by eschewing the role of parent. The requirement that they act as foster parents rather than parents may mean that fostering has to be recognized as a skilled and semi-professional task. The widespread reliance on the intuitive approach to foster care could be inappropriate in light of the changes in policy which have stressed the desirability of rehabilitation. This, and success as defined in this study, may be largely irreconcilable objectives unless some 'professionalization' of foster care takes place, and the foster parent role more clearly identified. Certainly the successful placements in this study could be charactierized as those in which circumstances favoured the development of a pseudo-adoptive situation: where the child had been placed young; where the foster parents were childless, or had no children near the age of the foster child, and so forth.

A somewhat similar hypothesis might be built up around the concept of conflict in the boarding-out situation: that the chances of success were, for example, a function of the level of conflict generated. Certainly it seems reasonable to suggest that conflict occurs between 'own' and foster children of rival ages. The foster mother would normally wish to be fair to the newcomer without penalizing her own offspring and this may also place her in a difficult position of conflict and vacillation. The particular problem which relationships between foster children and the children of the family may create is underlined by the fact that in those placements where there were only other foster children no significant tendency to failure was apparent. The fact that in something approaching 20 per cent of all the failures the adverse effect of the placement upon 'own' children was mentioned as one of the explicit reasons for removal also lends support to this thesis. In fact if the failures in foster families without 'own' children are excluded this proportion rises to 25 per cent. Perhaps in assessing the value of foster care some attention needs to be paid to the social 'costs' of 'own' children who become disturbed. When this happens foster parents may be placed in a position in which they are obliged to choose between the interests of their own families and the foster child. It is understandable that under such circumstances they ask for the foster child to be removed, albeit with genuine feelings of sorrow and regret.

Several commentators have pointed out that the foster child is also likely to face the problem of conflicting loyalties—loyalties to parents or foster parents; this home or that; these standards or those previously accepted. If this is the case, one might expect that the longer the child's experience of his own home and family, the more intense these conflicts. There was corroborative evidence for this assumption in the results of the study. For instance, the older the child at permanent separation from his mother, and the older at reception into care and subsequent fostering, the significantly less successful the placement.

Pursuing this thesis further a variety of circumstances may exist which could not only affect the degree of conflict but the ability of foster parents to tolerate or resolve it. Their motivation, skill, and the amount of help they receive will be important considerations. Time too may be on their side. The short-stay placement, for instance, may reach an apparently successful conclusion (child returned to parents) but might not have survived the strains for a longer period. In this study, as well as those of Gordon Trasler[1] and the Social Survey,[2] it was clear that the chance of failure mounted fairly rapidly to a peak somewhere about 18 months after the placement and then began to tail off steadily. The most likely time for a failure to occur seemed to be between 6 months and 2 years after placement. In this enquiry, for example, although the assessment period was stretched over 5 years, 50 per cent of the failures occurred during this 18-month

[1] Ibid., pp. 216 and 217.
[2] Ibid., p. 28.

period which only represents 30 per cent of the possible total risk period. It may be, therefore, that one of the ways of bearing conflict situations is knowing that there is a definite and predictable end in sight—not too far distant. One thinks of the foster mother unduly upset by being asked to keep a child a few weeks longer than expected.

The notions of role ambiguity and conflict could certainly form the bases for two interesting hypotheses. It is, of course, impossible to hope to fit all the results of this study into one comprehensive 'theory'—and one of the attractions of a predictive approach is that it relieves us from having to try. Nonetheless, a prediction study can suggest various possible hypotheses and the discussion of just two of these serves to illustrate the potentialities.

III

SPECIFIC AREAS FOR FUTURE STUDY

As well as suggesting more general hypotheses, this study highlighted a number of particular problems which might be examined further.[1] Some of them have already been touched upon elsewhere and arise directly from the results. Others are suggested either because they reflect important gaps in the information available, or because they became apparent as a result of a general concern with research in this field over several years.

In chapter 2 some of the difficulties encountered in defining success and failure were discussed. The criterion eventually chosen —whether or not the child stayed in his foster home—had certain advantages but was unable to take into account the practical possibilities available to the child care officers when the placements were made. In this sense it was somewhat detached from the administrative situation. Alternatively, however, the emphasis could have been placed upon evaluating the placement decision rather than the placement itself. This would have put the assessment firmly in the administrative setting. Instead of judging the placement against an ideal—whether this be permanency, adjustment in adult life, or whatever—this would entail

---

[1] For a general discussion of the sorts of question which can be asked most usefully in this general field see R. A. Parker's 'The Basis of Research in Adoption', *Case Conference*, Vol. 10, No. 4, September, 1963.

establishing whether the 'best' of a range of possible decisions had been made at the time. Although the outcome of such 'best' decisions may fall short of our ideal the placement decision could still rank as successful. Such an approach is different from that adopted in this study. It would, in the first place, be a more ambitious piece of research requiring considerably more resources, for it could only be done adequately by comparing not only the availability of alternatives but their eventual suitability: success in such an enquiry would always be relative. It is clear that this type of research is a crucial part of the evaluation of foster care and really calls for a general assessment of 'care' rather than one particular form of it. Similar problems arise in the study of sentencing. It is possible to study probation, for example, to see how successful this is with different sorts of offenders, but if we are concerned with the success of the sentence decision itself, then we must also study the effectiveness of the alternatives available to the magistracy—conditional discharge; fines; approved schools; fit person orders, and so forth.

This research also limited itself to the study of long-term placements. It has already been suggested earlier that differences exist between these placements and the growing number of short-term arrangements. In many ways the short-term placement is more difficult to evaluate: it hardly has time to establish clearly its success. There is also a singular lack of work done on the assessment of other forms of short-term care[1] and the critic may well ask whether the considerable demands made upon children's departments in arranging a two- or three-week foster placement are really justifiable. More study of the effect of different forms of short-term provision upon children needs to be undertaken before such critics can be answered with assurance. Certainly short periods of residential care appeared from this study not to affect adversely the chances of subsequent successful fostering. Research on the effects of institutional care has, in the past, been concerned predominantly with long periods of exposure and has tended to regard residential care as a basically similar experience for all children. Different ages may respond differently and the

[1] A major exception is of course the on-going study directed by Professor J. Tizard which, amongst other things, includes the examination of the effects of short-term residential care.

differences between Homes may now be as great as their similarities.

In the field of boarding-out it might be asked whether the foster
parents most suitable for long-term work are also suitable for
short-term placements. The results suggest that those who had
undertaken the care of one or two children for short periods
(presumably successfully) before a long-term placement were not
particularly successful. 'Trying out' foster parents on short-term
work may not, therefore, be justified or particularly helpful in
forecasting their success over a long period with one child. Again,
if there are differences between the abilities, motives and attitudes
of these two groups, then indiscriminate recruiting campaigns
might better be replaced by a two-pronged attack aimed at each
group separately.

It would be valuable if more research could be done in identify-
ing the differences (or establishing lack of difference) between the
long- and short-term fostering situation. The general recruitment
of foster parents too, needs further investigation—for if the choice
of foster parents is to be effectively increased many more need to
come forward to offer their services. What distinguishes those
who come forward from those who do not?[1] Recruitment campaigns are often disappointing in their results, perhaps, because
they are too indiscriminate in their appeal (advertising, in contrast, tends to aim at clearly definable groups: teenagers; house-
wives; smokers; pet-owners; car-owners, and so on). They may
also fail because they contain the implicit assumption that what is
stopping people from coming forward is lack of information.
In fact, from a small study recently undertaken,[2] it appeared that
the great majority of people interviewed were already remarkably
well-informed about the need for more foster parents and were
aware of the nature of foster care. Merely giving out more information seems, in light of this, an unlikely way of increasing
recruitment. It is noticeable how much more thought and money
goes into recruiting buyers for most consumer goods than has
ever been expended on this problem.

[1] This question is examined in a study undertaken by John Wakeford reported in the
British Journal of Sociology, Vol. XIV. No. 4, December, 1963.
[2] Unpublished study undertaken by Miss C. Collins, a student in the department of
Social Administration, London School of Economics.

In particular the part which payment to foster parents plays or can play in both recruitment and the clarification of their role and function warrants examination. If, as it has been suggested, the future of foster care is closely tied to its increasing professionalization, then adequate payment is one important element in its development. This is linked with the problem of organizing foster care. Today foster parents control 50 per cent of the resources for caring for deprived children; yet they remain largely outside and separate from the children's departments and societies. Optimum use of this form of care cannot be achieved, it might be suggested, unless foster parents can be used very much as if they were employees. If, for example, a foster mother is willing to act continuously in a short-term capacity, she needs to be 'on call'. Under these circumstances not only is a retaining fee reasonable but also such things as help with the cost of a telephone, together of course with generous payment which includes a fair element of reward. Organizations would be paying this not out of dewy-eyed sympathy, but for work done and as compensation for the foster parents' loss of autonomy. Foster parents will be paid to become part of the organization. Until this happens fostering will remain largely an important but nevertheless unpredictable part of the resources available for caring for children. If it does happen, child care officers may cease to feel indebted to foster parents and begin to achieve a relationship such as might be expected between professionals with somewhat different roles and skills which are nonetheless basically interdependent.

Other areas of study concerning the foster family which might well be pursued by a variety of different techniques are the relationships between children of the family and foster children, and the part played by foster fathers. Enough has already been said about the former, except to add that the attitudes of 'own' children to the arrangement might be revealing. Little information was available about the foster fathers in the records and there seems to have been a tendency to focus pre-eminently upon the foster mother-foster child relationship to the exclusion of various others which exist and may be influential. For instance, there was no attempt in this study to analyse the influence of the child's own parents upon the placement. Whilst in any case such information was not essential to its purpose, it would in addition have been difficult to determine. In general there seems to be a tendency for parents to express attitudes which favour their child going to residential care rather than a foster home: one wonders what part is played in subsequent success by parental commitment or opposition to the idea of a foster home for their child. If the child is to be 'severed' from its family this may not be too important. If, however, as is now the case, re-unification becomes the objective, it may matter very much. Certainly it would be valuable to have a systematic examination of the pattern and influence of parental visits to the foster homes.

On somewhat similar lines the impact of casework help and supervision obviously needs to be evaluated. For reasons explained in chapter 2[1] it was not attempted in this study. Like the problems of social work assessment in other fields,[2] this is a task beset with difficulties. One of these is that we are not in a position to offer this service to some and deny it to a control group. It might, however, be possible to evaluate the effects of more or less intensive casework help given to similar groups of foster homes. Even then, of course, it still remains difficult to judge what exactly is being offered the foster parents, and there may well be several different officers responsible for supervising a placement at different times. A tentative excursion was made in the study to investigate this issue. First, the average number of child care officers supervising each foster home throughout its duration was calculated: no significant difference emerged between successes and failures. Second, the frequency of visits was calculated as another crude measure of the intensity of help, but again no significant differences emerged. This is perhaps not surprising, for if a social worker has insufficient time to offer an intensive service to all those on her case load, she may use her skill in assessment of need to determine which are the weaker and less effective foster homes. As a result one suspects that a levelling-out process probably takes place whereby these weaker foster homes receive most help and the most competent (or those thought to be most able), the least.

[1] See p. 3.
[2] See for further discussion Gordon Rose 'Assessing the Results of Social Work', *Sociological Review*, Vol. 5, No. 2 (New Series), December, 1957.

Shifting the emphasis away from the foster home itself, there are several questions primarily concerning the children which could be usefully studied further. For instance, in this study 'behaviour problems' was treated very much as a homogeneous category, but the effect of different forms of disturbed behaviour upon fostering difficulties needs to be clarified. It was possible to show, for example, that enuresis was not likely to affect the placement adversely, and it seems too that physical handicaps proved no stumbling block to success. Clearly we need to know much more precisely the levels of tolerance and the amount of strain associated with different sorts of difficulty. A study relying exclusively upon recorded material is unlikely to be able to throw much light on such issues.

It was suggested earlier that the attitude of the child towards fostering may be important. Some children may not want to be fostered, possibly being aware of the inherent conflicts facing them in the situation.[1] In fact an 'institutional' setting, which is after all somewhat similar to the familiar school environment, may seem more attractive and less threatening. Such a thesis might well be studied in conjunction with what has appeared to be the problem of caring for both the bereaved child and the adolescent.

There may also be distinct differences between placements with relatives and those with strangers to be taken into account. Such a comparison was not possible in this study since placements with relatives were omitted. But since 8 per cent of all placements current in 1963 were with relatives, this is far from a negligible consideration: its study might indeed throw additional light on the whole boarding-out process. Similarly it was clear from their records that many of the children in the sample had been previously placed in private foster homes. The analysis of a wider sample of such arrangements, if these could be properly identified, might also provide interesting comparative data. In fact, do different 'sorts' of foster mothers undertake private work; do different 'sorts' of parents use them; are the problems in any way different, and just how extensive is this form of care?

These suggestions represent only a fraction of the many questions which could be usefully examined in the general field

[1] For example, see Janet Hitchman's novel, *King of the Barbareens*.

of foster care. There is no shortage of work to be done: amongst its other contributions each piece of research makes this increasingly clear, but at the same time helps us to formulate better the questions remaining unanswered. In many ways asking the right questions is the greatest single difficulty facing research. In this lies one of the crucial research skills. Poor questions can never be adequately compensated by sophisticated techniques or generous financial backing: in general they lead to disappointing results. Similarly, uninspired or conventional questions will only secure uninspired and conventional answers. Ideally, each piece of research should help us to ask better and more discriminating questions the next time.

IV

CONCLUSIONS

The study has not led us to any firm conclusions. This was not its aim. It was concerned with the construction of a statistical tool which would be a viable aid to social work practice. The results which were produced in developing the prediction table have also provided a basis for the discussion of many assumptions and theories about the dynamics of foster care. From this, however, a few conclusions can be made with some confidence, not because they represent facts discovered by this enquiry but because what was discovered was substantially supported by other previous work. It is the consensus of many findings which enables conclusions to be drawn and a beginning made with the construction of general theoretical frameworks. This process was well illustrated in John Bowlby's now famous monograph. Insufficient work has been done, however, on many aspects of foster care for such a stage to be reached, although reasonable concensus exists about three things. All are relatively simple and are perhaps already commonly accepted in the field. First, the age of the child is unanimously found to be a crucial factor; as far as fostering is concerned—the younger the better. A similar conclusion could probably also be drawn in the field of adoption. Second, the presence of children of the family about the age of the foster child is a situation likely to produce difficulty and needs to be treated with care. Third, children with behaviour disturbances are difficult to foster; though not necessarily children with physical handicaps. These may seem pedestrian conclusions: they are the only ones that can be confidently claimed at this stage.

However, from the standpoint of this study the principal conclusion is that predictive methods can be usefully employed and can offer a valuable means of making the results of research readily available in a practical form. Too often such methods have been regarded as inappropriate to the study of social work; largely because the legitimacy of the casework approach to the work itself has been carried over without sufficient consideration to the study of that work. It would be unfortunate, however, if the case study and statistical approaches were regarded as quite separate alternatives. The two methods should rather be thought of as complementary in both decision-making and research. In the latter field, for example, it may well prove most rewarding for those cases which are the exceptions to the general statistical pattern to be studied intensively by case study methods. It may be that it is from just such unique cases that most is learnt. Both approaches have their limitations and their weaknesses, but the weaknesses of one tend to be the strong-points of the other.

As in all research a final plea must be made for more studies employing a variety of methods and asking a whole range of questions. Perhaps progress will be made with the facilities for financing research which the 1963 Children and Young Persons Act provides. For the sake of the children involved one hopes so.

———

ADDITIONAL STATISTICS ON THE CHILD CARE SERVICE

A BRIEF outline of the 'form' of the child care service was provided in chapter 1. Some additional statistics serve to describe more fully its 'content' and to underline some of the changes taking place since 1948. The principal sources from which these figures have been taken are the annual statistical returns *Children in the Care of Local Authorities in England and Wales,* which have been published by the Home Office since 1952, and the Sixth, Seventh, and Eighth reports of the work of the Children's Department also published by the Home Office.

TABLE 1

Total number of children in care of local authorities in England and Wales, 1949–1963 and the numbers per 1,000 of the population under 18; proportion in care as a result of fit person orders; and the proportion of boys

	No.	No. per 1,000	% F.P.O.	% Boys
Nov. 1949	55,255		25·4	55·5
Nov. 1950	58,987		26·4	55·4
Nov. 1951	62,691		27·3	—
Nov. 1952	64,682	5·6	28·5	55·2
Nov. 1953	65,309	6·2	29·2	55·5
Nov. 1954	64,560	5·5	29·6	55·5
Mar. 1956	62,347	5·3	30·0	55·5
Mar. 1957	62,033	5·2	29·5	55·6
Mar. 1958	62,070	5·5	29·6	55·5
Mar. 1959	61,580	5·1	30·1	55·5
Mar. 1960	61,729	5·0	30·6	55·2

Mar. 1961	62,199	5·0	31·4	55·2
Mar. 1962	63,648	5·1	32·2	55·0
Mar. 1963	64,807	5·1	32·8	54·8

Source: Figures for 1949–51 are given on p. 2 of the statistical return for 1952; for 1952 onwards they are taken from the annual returns:

1952	Cmnd. 8910	1959	Cmnd. 914
1953	Cmnd. 9145	1960	Cmnd. 1237
1954	Cmnd. 9488	1961	Cmnd. 1599
1956	Cmnd. 9881	1962	Cmnd. 1876
1957	Cmnd. 411	1963	Cmnd. 2240
1958	Cmnd. 632		

These basic figures and the various proportions have been fairly steady over the fourteen years. The number in care on fit person orders has been rising gradually every year, but the proportion of boys to girls in care remains remarkably constant.

The distribution of children in care by age groups (table 2), also remained fairly steady, although in recent years there has been a slight increase in the proportion of 'under 2s' and a slight decline in those of school age. Unfortunately the 5–15 group is too wide: were it further broken down some other variations might have been revealed over the years.

TABLE 2

The Age Grouping of Children in Care of Local Authorities in England and Wales

	Under 2 %	2 under 5 %	5 under 15 %	15 & over %
Nov. 1952	6·5	13·8	62·4	17·3
Nov. 1953	6·3	13·2	62·2	18·3
Nov. 1954	5·8	13·0	62·0	19·2
Mar. 1956	5·8	12·1	62·0	20·1
Mar. 1957	6·3	11·9	61·6	20·2
Mar. 1958	6·2	12·0	61·4	20·4
Mar. 1959	6·3	11·9	60·7	21·1
Mar. 1960	6·5	12·3	59·7	21·5
Mar. 1961	6·8	12·1	59·4	21·7
Mar. 1962	7·5	12·4	59·0	21·1
Mar. 1963	7·8	12·7	58·7	20·8

Source: The annual statistical summaries 1952–63.
Note: Proportions, as in the preceding chapters, add to a total of 100 per cent horizontally.

TABLE 3

Manner of Accommodation of Children in Care³—England and Wales, 1952–63

	Mar. 1963	Mar. 1962	Mar. 1961	Mar. 1960	Mar. 1959	Mar. 1958	Mar. 1957	Mar. 1956	Nov. 1954	Nov. 1953	Nov. 1952
	%	%	%	%	%	%	%	%	%	%	%
Boarded-out with non-relative²	40·3	39·5	38·5	37·9	36·7	34·6	34·6	34·3	} 44·5	} 42·2	} 40·6
Boarded-out with relative¹ ²	7·9	8·0	8·2	8·6	9·0	9·4	9·3	9·2			
In Lodgings²	1·7	1·5	1·6	1·6	1·5	1·4	1·4	1·6			
In Residential Employment²	1·1	1·2	1·2	1·2	1·4	1·5	1·8	2·1			
Local Authority Nursery	5·0	5·3	5·5	5·7	5·9	6·5	6·8	7·1	7·5	7·9	7·8
Reception Homes	2·5	2·4	2·5	2·6	2·4	2·5	2·3	2·3	1·7	1·6	1·8
Family Group Homes⁴	9·1	8·9	8·5	8·2	8·1	8·0	7·5	6·6	5·6	5·6	6·5
Other L.A. Children's Homes	13·3	14·1	14·9	15·5	16·0	17·3	17·5	18·7	21·5	22·5	22·4
Residential Provision for the Handicapped	2·9	2·9	3·3	3·6	3·5	3·7	3·9	3·5	3·6	3·4	3·1
Hostels	1·6	1·6	1·6	1·5	1·8	1·8	1·9	1·8	1·8	1·6	1·6
Voluntary Homes	5·7	5·8	5·8	6·2	6·6	6·9	7·0	7·4	8·2	9·4	10·1
Home on Trial⁵	4·6	4·1	} 8·4	{ 3·2	7·1	6·4	6·0	5·4	5·6	5·8	6·1
Other	4·3	4·7		4·2							
	100·0	100·0	100·0	100·0	100·0	100·0	100·0	100·0	100·0	100·0	100·0

Source: Annual Statistical Returns and the Eighth Report.

(See facing page for footnotes).

The two principal methods of accommodating children who are received into the care of local authorities are either boarding-out or placement in residential establishments of some sort. There has been a gradual increase in the proportion of children boarded-out or placed in family group homes in England and Wales and a gradual decline in the proportion in larger local authority homes, residential nurseries, or voluntary homes. This pattern can be seen in table 3. In addition it is interesting to see that although the proportion boarded-out continues to rise slowly the proportion placed with relatives is becoming smaller.

[1] From the 1956 return onwards it was possible to see how many children were in fact boarded-out with relatives. This information is given in note 2 to table 1 of the returns. Of those boarded-out in the years 1956–63 the following proportions were with relatives:

	%		%
1956	21·2	1960	18·5
1957	21·1	1961	17·6
1958	21·2	1962	16·8
1959	19·6	1963	16·5

Of those children boarded-out with relatives, in each year the following proportions were already in that home when 'boarded-out' officially:

	%		%
1956	63·5	1960	65·0
1957	64·7	1961	62·0
1958	65·1	1962	59·1
1959	64·4	1963	60·0

[2] These categories were all reported as 'boarded-out' until March 1956. This is clear from table 1 (p. 101) in the 8th Report of the Work of the Children's Department, 1961.

[3] From March 1956 the base for the calculation of the proportion of children accommodated in different ways—given in table 2 of the annual returns—was modified. Between 1956 and 1961 children in residential employment or lodgings were deducted from the total of children in care (footnote to table 2 of annual reports of that period). There seems no good reason for this except that the proportions boarded-out appeared to rise more than they actually did. The proportions in table 3 above have not made this deduction and hence do not compare exactly with proportions given in the annual returns. From 1962 onwards those children 'home on trial' were also deducted from the total in care before percentages boarded-out etc., were calculated. Unhappily no base is given for the calculation of percentages in their table 2 after 1961.

[4] From 1956 onwards this classification was no longer used—a new one was introduced 'Homes for not more than 12 children', which would appear to be very similar.

[5] Figures for 'home on trial' in 1962 and 1963 have been deduced and percentages worked accordingly. Since for example in the 1963 return the proportion boarded-out is given as 52·0 per cent and this has been calculated on the base of the total children in care less those in lodgings, in residential employment, and home on trial and figures for those in lodgings and residential employment are given, the number home on trial is arrived at by solving the equation: $\dfrac{x}{n - (a + b + c)} = 0·52$ where x is the number boarded-out; n the actual total number in care; a the number in lodgings; b the number in residential employment and c (the unknown) those home on trial. For 1960 the actual figure is provided in the 8th Report, table 1, p. 101.

These figures have been further analysed by sex in the returns. The break-down by the sex of those boarded-out is particularly of interest. This is given in table 4.

TABLE 4

Percentage of Children Boarded-out in England and Wales Analysed by their Sex

	Boys %	Girls %	Total %
Nov. 1949	29	41	35
Nov. 1950	31	43	37
Nov. 1952	35	47	41
Nov. 1953	37	49	42
Nov. 1954	39	51	44
Mar. 1956	40	51	45
Mar. 1957	40	52	45
Mar. 1958	41	51	46
Mar. 1959	41	51	46
Mar. 1960	42	52	46
Mar. 1961	42	52	47
Mar. 1962	43	53	47
Mar. 1963	44	53	48

Source: 1949   Sixth Report, page 9.
        1950   Seventh Report, page 153.
        1952–63 Annual returns.

The increase in the proportion of children boarded-out appears both in the case of the boys and the girls, but it is clear that a larger proportion of the girls than the boys are boarded-out. The increase in the proportion of children in care who were boarded-out occurred primarily between 1949 and 1954.

APPENDIX II

SUPPLEMENTARY DEFINITIONS

1. *'Long-term'*

Long-term placements were defined as follows:

(i) If it was stated in the case records before placement that it was to be long-term it was classed as such, unless this was specifically corrected later before a breakdown occurred.

(ii) However, if it was stated on the case record before placement that it was to be for a holiday, emergency, trial or short-term only and the child was removed from the home at the end of such a period, then that placement was considered short-term and excluded from the sample.

(iii) If such an initial placement developed into a long-term one (i.e. it was stated to have become so in the records), then it was included as a long-term placement and reckoned to have run from the first date of boarding-out.

(iv) However briefly the placement lasted, if it was considered to be long-term before the boarding-out or classed as such after being made but before failure, it was nevertheless included in the sample as a long-term placement.

(v) If there was no mention of either long- or short-term placement anywhere in the record a pragmatic criterion was adopted: if the child had been in the foster home more than a year it was classed as long-term. This possibly introduced a bias in the sample in favour of successes, since if a child was boarded-out long-term and this was nowhere mentioned and he failed under a year, he would have been excluded as an apparent short-term placement. However, there were very few cases indeed which had to be classified in this fashion. The previous four criteria sufficed for the great majority.

2. *'Close relatives'*:

Close relatives of the child included maternal or paternal aunts

ACKNOWLEDGEMENTS

I WOULD like to express my thanks to a number of people who have generously given assistance and advice in the course of this study. I am indebted to the Children's Committee of the Kent County Council for allowing me to conduct the research in their area and to have access to the necessary case records. In particular I would like to thank the Children's Officer, Miss D. E. Harvie, and the many members of the department who gave me a great deal of help.

I am very grateful too for the advice and help given me throughout this study by Professor D. V. Donnison and for the encouragement of Professor R. M. Titmuss. I have also appreciated the advice of Mr L. T. Wilkins and Dr M. H. Quenouille in regard to the statistical aspects of the enquiry. Robin Huws Jones read the draft and amongst other things, helped me to avoid including several passages which were not clear. Of course I alone am responsible for any shortcomings or inaccuracies which may appear in the book.

The research would never have been completed had it not been for the aid of a generous grant from the Sir Halley Stewart Trust and for this I am especially grateful. They have also contributed generously to part of the cost of publication. Thanks are also due to the London School of Economics who awarded me a research bursary; to the University of London Central Research Fund and the department of Social Administration at the School of Economics for grants for certain specific expenses.

(ii) If this was *not* a sufficient criterion then a second was invoked. When the child continued to have regular holidays with the foster parents and there was no indication of failure before the child left the foster home, it was classed as a success. If *no* further holidays were spent in the foster home, the case was classed as a failure.

APPENDIX III

NOTES ON STATISTICAL METHOD

OVER thirty factors were discussed in chapters 4 and 5; others of less general interest were not mentioned. Together, however, these represent the material which forms the basis for the multivariate analysis and from which the prediction table must be constructed. However, a very large number of factors is difficult to manipulate. Consequently it was decided that before the analysis was commenced some *a priori* reduction of the number of variables would have to be made. A convenient, though not entirely satisfactory way of doing this is to employ tests of significance, on the assumption that if a factor is not significantly associated with the criterion in its zero order form it will be unlikely to make a useful contribution to the discrimination after it has been studied in its multivariate context. Arbitrarily, only those factors were taken into the analysis which reached a 5 per cent level of significance. The analysis thus became a much more manageable problem and it is doubtful whether any factors which could have contributed significantly to accounting for the variation between the successes and failures were excluded. Mannheim and Wilkins made a similar *a priori* reduction in their study by including in the final analysis only those items which had reached a $2\frac{1}{2}$ per cent level of significance in their zero order form.

A further limitation was placed on the 'input' information at this stage because of the adoption of a simple solution to the problem of dealing with dichotomous and continuous variables in the same analysis. Throughout, this problem was overcome by treating all continuous factors as if they were dichotomous; that is, by combining the various frequency classes in such a way that there were only two possible classifications, e.g. 'had or had not', 'below and above a certain point', and so on. These combinations on either side of a cutting point were made in such a way that the successes on one side and the failures on the other side were maximized. Clearly some precision is sacrificed in this procedure. The accuracy of the final prediction table may be diminished, and the validation study may appear less impressive because this process of 'dichotomizing' is somewhat arbitrary. A slightly different choice of the point at which a division of each continuous variable was made might have been more appropriate for general applicability.

Initially then the multivariate analysis had to take into account 14 dichotomous variables; demonstrate their interrelationship; indicate which were to be rejected and which retained for use in a final prediction table, and attach relevant weights to each. This problem is basically one of predicting an unknown variable from others with known values, and is very similar to a regression problem. The 'best' prediction was in fact obtained by solving a set of multiple regression equations. The particular method adopted is discussed in M. H. Quenouille's *Associated Measurement* and the reader is referred to this. For those more specifically interested in the detailed statistical basis of this study, a duplicated paper has been produced and is obtainable upon request from:

> The National Institute for Social Work Training,
> Mary Ward House,
> 5–7, Tavistock Place,
> London, W.C.1.

Such technical details have not been included in either the main text or this appendix because it was felt they were not of sufficient general interest.

APPENDIX IV

MATRIX OF CONCOMITANCE

In looking at the network of interrelationships amongst the factors considered in this study it is valuable to be able to see the total picture without undue difficulty. A useful method of doing this in a quickly comprehensible manner is the matrix of concomitance. The principles upon which its construction rests have been fully described in J. P. Martin's *Social Aspects of Prescribing*. In brief it provides a summary of the degree of association between any one factor and others.

The factors included in the matrix below are those which reached a 5 per cent level of significance in their zero order form, together with certain others of more general interest such as sex; whether the child was in care under the Children Act or on a fit person order; year of placement, and so forth. It would make the matrix unnecessary to comment on all the relationships but it is worth pointing out first that the relationships can be in either direction (A can be associated with B or alternatively with *not*-B). Such direction is shown by the use of the symbol N in the cells. Where this appears the relationship is negative: where it does not appear the relationship is positive. It may also be useful to draw the reader's attention to the importance in some cases of lack of significant relationship, and to explain why the year of placement has been included. In a way this is an artificial variable which was adopted in order to see whether there were any significant differences between the two years of placement (1952 and 1953) used in the sample. If considerable differences were found it would tend to suggest either that something was amiss with the sample or else that the problem varied drastically from one year to another. It can be seen that the results with this factor were satisfactory, there being only two factors (9 and 16) which reached the 5 per cent level.

MATRIX OF CONCOMITANCE

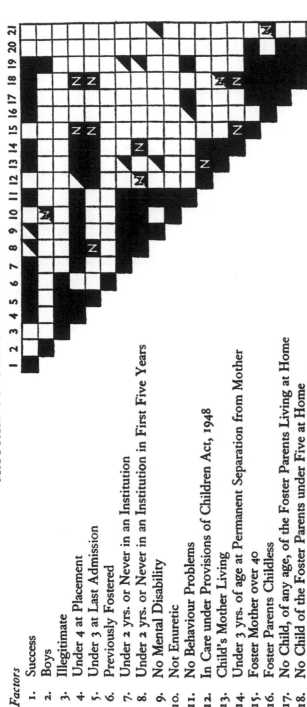

Factors

1. Success
2. Boys
3. Illegitimate
4. Under 4 at Placement
5. Under 3 at Last Admission
6. Previously Fostered
7. Under 2 yrs. or Never in an Institution
8. Under 2 yrs. or Never in an Institution in First Five Years
9. No Mental Disability
10. Not Enuretic
11. No Behaviour Problems
12. In Care under Provisions of Children Act, 1948
13. Child's Mother Living
14. Under 3 yrs. of age at Permanent Separation from Mother
15. Foster Mother over 40
16. Foster Parents Childless
17. No Child, of any age, of the Foster Parents Living at Home
18. No Child of the Foster Parents under Five at Home
19. No Child of the Foster Parents within 5 yrs. of the Placed Child
20. Foster Mother had already been Foster Mother for more than a year
21. Year of Placement 1952

Notes: ◩ ▦ = significant at 5 per cent level (P<0·05)
■ = significant at 1 per cent level (P<0·01)

Where N is written into the cell the significant association is negative.

BIBLIOGRAPHY

Accord, The Journal of the Association of Child Care Officers.

Association of Children's Officers, *Proceedings of the Annual Conferences*.

Baxter, Adah, 'The Adjustment of Children to Foster Homes'. *Smiths College Studies in Social Work*, Vol. 7, No. 3, March, 1937.

Baylor, E. N. and Monachesi, Elio. D., *Rehabilitation of Children*. Harper, New York, 1939.

Bowlby, John, *Maternal Care and Mental Health*. W.H.O. Monograph Series, No. 2, 1951.

Bross, Erwin D. J., *Design for Decision*. Macmillan, New York, 1953.

Burlingham, Dorothy and Freud, Anna, *Annual Report of a Residential War Nursery*. 1942.

Charnley, Jean, *The Art of Child Placement*. Minneapolis, University of Minnesota, 1955.

Donnison, D. V., *The Neglected Child and Social Services*, Manchester University Press, 1954.
Social Policy and Administration (National Institute for Social Work Training Series), Allen and Unwin, 1965.

Dudley, Virginia, 'Foster Mothers: Successful and Unsuccessful', *Smiths College Studies in Social Work*, Vol. III, No. 2, December, 1932.

Dyson, D. M., *The Foster Home and the Boarded-out Child*. Allen and Unwin, 1947.

General Register Office, *Census of England and Wales, 1951*, County Report, Kent. H.M.S.O.

Glass, D. V., 'The Application of Social Research'. *British Journal of Sociology*, Vol. I, No. 1, March, 1950.

Glueck, Eleanor T., 'Predicting Juvenile Delinquency'. *British Journal of Delinquency*, No. 4, April 1952.

Goldfarb, William, 'Infant Rearing as a Factor in Foster Home

Placement'. *American Journal of Orthopsychiatry*, Vol. XIV, No. 1, January, 1944.

'Infant Rearing and Problem Behaviour', *American Journal of Orthopsychiatry*, Vol. XIII, No. 2, April, 1943.

Gray, P. G. and Parr, Elizabeth A., *Children in Care and the Recruitment of Foster Parents*. Social Survey, S.S. 249. November, 1957.

Healy, William, Bronner, Augusta, Baylor, E. M., and Murphy, J. P., *Reconstructing behaviour in Youth*. Judge Baker Foundation Publication No. 5, Knopf, New York, 1927.

Heywood, J. S., *Children in Care*. Routledge and Kegan Paul, 1959.

Hitchman, Janet, *King of the Barbareens*.

Home Office, Sixth Report of the Work of the Children's Department, H.M.S.O., May 1951.

Seventh Report of the Work of the Children's Department, H.M.S.O., November, 1955.

Eighth Report of the Work of the Children's Department, H.M.S.O. 1961.

Memorandum—Departmental Reply to the Sixth Report from the Select Committee on Estimates. Session 1951–2 (Child Care), 1952.

Memorandum on the Care of Children under Five Years of Age. 1955.

Circular No. 258/1952.

Memorandum on the Boarding-Out of Children Regulations. 1955.

Children in the Care of Local Authorities in England and Wales. (Annual Returns, commencing 1952).

Home Office and Ministry of Health, Joint Memorandum on the Boarding-out of Children and Young Persons. 1946.

House of Commons, Sixth Report from the Select Committee on Estimates, 1951/2 (Child Care)—235.

Isaacs, Susan (Ed.), *The Cambridge Evacuation Survey*. Methuen, 1941.

Kent County Council, Children's Committee. Reports 1948/50, 1950/3, 1953/58.

Lewis, Hilda, *Deprived Children*. Oxford University Press, 1954.

Lowrey, L. G., 'Personality Distortion in Early Institutional Care'. *American Journal of Orthopsychiatry*, Vol. X, 1940.

Mannheim, H. and Wilkins, L. T., *Prediction Methods in Relation to Borstal Training*. H.M.S.O. 1954.

Martin, J. P., *Social Aspects of Prescribing*. Heinemann, 1958.

Meyer, H. J., Jones, W., and Borgatta, E. F., 'The Decision of Unmarried Mothers to keep or Surrender their Babies'. *Social Work* (Journal of the National Association of Social Workers), Vol. I, No. 2, April, 1956.

Monachesi, Elio D., 'An Evaluation of Recent Major Efforts at Prediction'. *American Journal of Sociology*, Vol. VI, 1941.

Mordy, Isobel, *The Child needs a Home*. Harrap, 1956.

National Council for the Unmarried Mother and Her Child, *Classified Bibliography on Illegitimacy*, 1958.

Parker, R. A., 'The Basis of Research in Adoption', *Case Conference*, Vol. 10, No. 4, September, 1963.

Quenouille, M. H., *Associated Measurement*. Butterworth, 1952.

Report on the 'Circumstances which led to the Boarding-Out of Dennis and Terence O'Neill at Bank Farm, Minsterley, and the steps taken to supervise their welfare'. Cmd. 6636, 1945. H.M.S.O. (Monckton).

Report of the Care of Children Committee, Cmd. 6922, 1946. H.M.S.O. (Curtis).

Report of the Committee on Homeless Children, Cmd. 6911, 1946. H.M.S.O. (Clyde).

Rose, Gordon, 'Assessing the Results of Social Work'. *Sociological Review*, Vol. 5, No. 2, (New Series), December, 1957.

Scottish Advisory Council on Child Care, Report of the Boarding-out Committee, 1950.

Scottish Home Department, *Children in Care of Local Authorities in Scotland*. (Annual Returns commencing 1957).

Simon, Abraham J., 'Social and Psychological Factors in Child Placement', *American Journal of Orthopsychiatry*, Vol. XX, No. 2, April, 1950.

Simon, H. A., *Administrative Behaviour*. Macmillan, New York, (2nd Edition), 1961.

Stroud, J., *The Shorn Lamb*, Penguin Books, 1962.

Theis, Sophie van Senden, *How Foster Children Turn Out*. (Study made for the State Charities Association—No. 165), New York, 1924.

Titmuss, R. M., *Problems of Social Policy*. H.M.S.O., 1950.

Trasler, G. B., *Foster Home Success and Failure*. Thesis for Ph.D., London, 1955.

In Place of Parents. Routledge and Kegan Paul, 1960.

Wakeford, J., 'Fostering—a Sociological Perspective', *British Journal of Sociology*, Vol. XIV, No. 4, December, 1963.

Wilkins, L. T., 'Some Developments in Prediction Methodology in Applied Social Research', *British Journal of Sociology*, Vol. VI, No. 4, December, 1955.

Wootton, Barbara, *Social Science and Social Pathology*. Allen and Unwin, 1959.

INDEX

INDEX OF PERSONS

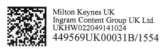